The Ceiling Outside

Also by Noga Arikha

Passions and Tempers: A History of the Humours

Napoleon and the Rebel:
A Story of Brotherhood, Passion, and Power
(*with Marcello Simonetta*)

The Ceiling Outside

The Science and Experience of the Disrupted Mind

NOGA ARIKHA

BASIC BOOKS

New York

In memoriam
Anne Atik Arikha (1932–2021)

To the WoWs

Basic Books
Hachette Book Group
1290 Avenue of the Americas, New York, NY 10104
www.basicbooks.com

Printed in the United States of America

Originally published in 2022 in Great Britain by Basic Books London
First US Edition: May 2022

Published by Basic Books, an imprint of Perseus Books, LLC, a subsidiary of Hachette Book Group, Inc. The Basic Books name and logo is a trademark of the Hachette Book Group.

The Hachette Speakers Bureau provides a wide range of authors for speaking events. To find out more, go to www.hachettespeakersbureau.com or call (866) 376-6591.

The publisher is not responsible for websites (or their content) that are not owned by the publisher.

Typeset in Janson Text by Palimpsest Book Production Ltd, Falkirk, Stirlingshire

Library of Congress Control Number: 2021950279

ISBNs: 9781541600874 (hardcover); 9781541600881 (ebook)

LSC-C

Printing 1, 2022

Contents

The main character is always the hardest work.
Deborah Levy, *The Cost of Living* (2018)

What was life, really? It was warmth, the warmth produced by instability attempting to preserve form, a fever of matter that accompanies the ceaseless dissolution and renewal of protein molecules, themselves transient in their complex and intricate construction. It was the existence of what, in actuality, has no inherent ability to exist, but only balances with sweet, painful precariousness on one point of existence in the midst of this feverish, interwoven process of decay and repair.
Thomas Mann, *The Magic Mountain* (1924)
trans. John E. Woods (1995)

I

The Double Mirror

At the still point of the turning world. Neither
    flesh nor fleshless;
Neither from nor towards; at the still point, there
    the dance is,
But neither arrest nor movement. And do not call
    it fixity,
Where past and future are gathered. Neither
    movement from nor towards,
Neither ascent nor decline. Except for the point,
    the still point,
There would be no dance, and there is only the
    dance.

T. S. Eliot, *Four Quartets*,
from 'Burnt Norton', II

Did you call me?

No, Mummy, you called me.

Well, the phone rang and you hung up and I just answered.
Are you in Paris?

Yes, you called me in Paris.

I need your help, urgently, I need you to give me your
phone number, I can't find it.

But Mummy you just called me!

Oh yes that's right. How are the children?

And how old is the eldest, and which one is he. And all these people are coming over tonight, there is a committee, but I must call them, I don't find their phone numbers. And there is a review of my book on the front page of the magazine, I can't remember the name of it. And it must be my mother who gave me this beautiful scarf.

But Mummy she died in 1986.

Did she?

Yes, she did, and she could hardly have bought such an elegant scarf in her religious neighbourhood in Jerusalem.

Well, you never know, she could have, people bought all sorts of things! And I must call her.

And on it goes. Memory chopped up into incoherent bits. Sentences that don't stick together while the syntax is perfect. Past, present, future, all neatly separated – but what goes into which, no longer. All is mixed up. Names, children and grand-children, episodes, sounds – familiarity disintegrating. Stories un-told and transposed from one place, one face, to another. Coherence and incoherence coexisting, akin to the sane and the mad rubbing shoulders over drinks at a cocktail party. The happy hour. The eleventh hour. The evening of existence almost spent while joy overtakes melancholy and a strange calm replaces anxiety. She frets less, laughs more, enjoys life and feels young and alive; her jokes are funnier than ever, their associations free and wild. Her sayings are somehow sensical and they can be double-edged. 'Just have fun! they said with tears in their eyes,' was one. Her memory is shunting her from place to place, as if she were ice-skating blindfolded, while the only way for us to remain in our place is not to follow her, to ignore, to let go, let her go, let it be, let it unfold, and occasionally take notes. We can only be good daughters by not being the daughters we once were. We take it in. We must laugh. She is not sad. We cannot be sad either. 'The ceiling inside, the ceiling outside,' she said the other day, sing-song and amused.

No one can do anything much about dementia, so far. Our mother Anne Atik is a poet. Or rather, was a poet. A reader, who emerged out of her religious upbringing in Brooklyn through a passion for Jane Austen, the Brontës, poetry and music. At the time I wrote the lines above, caught within the urgent, fleeting, incomprehensible present of it all, she was still able, when she came for dinner, slowly to read children's books and programmes of local activities, in thrall to how interesting they were. The *TLS* still piled up by her bedside, along with various novels and essays she had been reading over the past year. She had started writing her memoir some years before, about her childhood, youth, marriage to our father, the painter and survivor Avigdor Arikha, friendships, especially with 'Sam' – Beckett – about whom she had written a marvellous book, called *How it Was*, published two decades before. But she already had little memory left. She said then that, yes, she was writing. I knew she was not. At the time, at least, she still remembered that some writing was supposed to be going on. When I asked her one day, 'Are you writing your memoir?' she said, 'What's left of it.' By now, she has forgotten that too.

I had no idea when I embarked on this book, which features people I had never met before and would never see again, that our mother would take her place within its pages. I could not have known then that I would experience from close up how, in the space of a few months, so much of what makes up the life of a person can disintegrate. She was fine, or ordinarily anxious, when I started. She was indeed writing her memoir. But her computer desktop had become a mighty mess, she often was confused and erratic, and we knew something was amiss. By the time I had finished my second draft, she no longer could use the computer. She needed full-time care. Her friends, especially the young writers who admired her, still visit. She still sees my sister Alba and me as her daughters. But she is no longer the interlocutor we had known.

As I write these lines now, she has forgotten I have been writing a book based on patients of a neuropsychiatry unit at the Pitié-Salpêtrière hospital in Paris, the very place where, it so happens, she consults her neurologist every few months – each time marvelling more at the beauty of everything and at how very happy she is. One day, before dementia had clearly asserted itself, we travelled together to London on the Eurostar – it would turn out to be her last ever trip on that train, to the city she loved so much – and she read on my open laptop the chapter about the first patient I wrote about, a young woman who experiences amnesia. I remember feeling, and then suppressing, a terrible sense of irony. An irony I would be forced to contend with often as I reworked the book, thinking again about all the patients I had so fleetingly seen.

Those many other stories of unravelling I was privy to at the hospital, some of which you will read here, have indeed taken on new meaning. The present and the personal have somehow inserted themselves into this book, the theme of which is the nature of the self. Not myself. Not herself. The human self in general, as studied by science, understood throughout history, and analysed by philosophy. The self that the scientist, historian, philosopher tend to set aside as they think about other selves. And the book is still about all this. But life can interrupt one's best efforts at contemplating it from a safe distance.

The Pitié-Salpêtrière hospital happens to be quite close to the flat where, for now, my mother still lives, and where Alba and I grew up. And the story of how I came to be interested in what the self is begins here, in my childhood home. I was about ten years old, the age of my eldest son as I write this now. A family friend whose identity I have long forgotten gave my mother a thick, laminated, blue kitchen apron. I still see the apron clearly, and remember where it hung in the rather shabby kitchen of those days. A white curly-haired dog, who looked a bit like Snoopy, was framed by three yellow comic strip squares containing thought bubbles. I remember exactly the writing in the bubbles. Square one: 'I think, therefore I am.' Square two: 'But if I only think I think, how do I know I think?' Square three: 'I mean, I could only be thinking I think . . . I think . . . I think . . .' Suddenly, it occurred to me that one could think about thinking. It was like the double mirror that lined the entrance hall of our building, and in which one found oneself reflected infinitely, with no horizon in view, all the way to the unthinkable. The double mirror was the thinking self, then, also reflected to infinity. Who was the thinker? How did thinking work?

It was a vertiginous view for a ten-year-old which triggered vertiginous questions about who I was as a being who could think about herself thinking. A being who was a thinking self – that is, a being *aware* of being a thinking self who could think about herself as a thinking self, *aware of being aware* of it, *ad infinitum* as in those facing mirrors. Most of us, once grown up, will have forgotten what it is like to experience this dawning of self-consciousness when we *become* aware of being aware, because we only start forming long-term memories as we develop this awareness.[1] And once grown up, we also take for granted our daily use of our rational abilities – those that, for instance, enable me to compose these words and you to read, comprehend and consider them. I, for one, never stopped wondering about this awareness. And by reading about the dog and the mirrors, you may suddenly have become aware of your ability to think about these abilities. Just as I have become acutely aware, watching my mother, that these abilities can disintegrate.

At the best of times, our very awareness – of ourselves and of the world – is fluctuating. We feel as much as we think. Feeling and thinking are intertwined, the one feeding into the other. We can feel a thought and think about an emotion. Our mental life is in fact not stable. We usually know what we feel, but sometimes we can become confused about our feelings. Sometimes we may panic, at others we may be overwhelmed by despair or sadness. We may lose cognitive capacities, or forget parts of our lives – as is happening to my mother. When the human mind veers off course in this way, away from cognitive clarity, it exposes some of its mechanisms to the clinicians – neurologists and psychiatrists – who try to identify the problem and where possible help get us back on track, if we choose, or are impelled, to seek medical care, thereby becoming patients. Scientists who study the mind, such as psychologists and neuroscientists, help us understand how feeling and thinking work.

So this book is about both the self as it *studies* itself, and the self as it *loses* itself. Its starting premise, which is not as evident as it may seem, is that the sense of self is profoundly anchored in our body. I want to bring to the fore how this is – how we cannot understand the self without the brain or the brain without the body that it serves. Nor does this embodied self exist without other people. Whatever the labels we use to describe the ailments afflicting patients whose minds have veered off course, we can only treat people effectively, with empathy and with dignity, if we recognize that the person is not reducible to the brain, or to the ailments afflicting it.

This book explores what science and medicine can reveal about the embodied self, along the continuum of health and illness. A state of health and well-being, one could say, is one in which we do not need to think about our embodied organism in any way other than the sensorial pleasures it affords, where we are immersed within our environment, engaged in an activity, involved with others. Illness, be it physical or emotional pain, affects the very foundation on which the sense of self we otherwise take for granted rests: what we feel ourselves to be can be upended. Yet there is a long gradation between one state and the other. There are the neurological illnesses such as the one afflicting my mother, which suppress even the awareness of illness, and which do not result in a clear sense of pain, or in an awareness of a lost sense of self. And there are others where the sufferer is aware that something is wrong, reminding us that what we feel ourselves to be is in fact constructed. We may experience the construction blocks falling apart but what we rarely realize within our own experience is that how we exist as embodied selves is a highly complex business involving the brain and body engaged in constant interaction.

Some scientists are studying what it takes for this subjective experience to happen, but these studies are not yet widely known to the general public, and this view of the self as embodied is by no means mainstream even within the neurosciences. Nor has it yet fully made its way into the consulting rooms of mainstream neurology and psychiatry – it is central mostly to body-centred practices, from yoga and meditation to osteopathy. Yet I believe it is a wise starting point for an investigation of the mind, and of mental health. As we will see, this view has consequences for our understanding of how we fall ill and how we can get better, and also of how we make decisions, how we process our emotions, how we understand each other, and how we relate to each other in private as well as in society at large and even between peoples.

The book is therefore also about boundaries: those within which science can answer questions such as those asked by the dog on that apron; those within which it is possible for medicine to improve a confused person's life; and those within which we define illness and health. These boundaries emerge most clearly when we take a historical and anthropological step away from the here and now. An awareness of how our explanations change with time, and within and across cultures, helps us make better use of the ones we have today: indeed, assumptions about the nature of illness or what is normal behaviour, and about what happens to a person afflicted with dementia, are products of cultures, societies and their histories.

Whether they can ever be answered or not, questions are a good place to begin an exploration. And I date my wish to understand what it means to be a self-conscious being – to be a 'thinker' thinking about thought – to the arrival of that apron. At the age of ten I had little idea of what philosophy was, or that many people worldwide were invested in looking past the double mirror and researching consciousness – that there existed psychology and related sciences of mind. And I did not know that the apron quoted the seventeenth-century French philosopher René Descartes, whose native country I was living in. But I would find out, in time. For I studied philosophy in high school (as one does in France), and then at university in London. And I eventually understood how, through versions of his famous statement, 'I think, therefore I am,' Descartes established that our very awareness of being a thinking person was what guaranteed that our knowledge about the world was true. The ability to think was a demonstration of the reality of thought, self, and world. Mind – or soul, as one called it at the time – was necessarily conscious, and entailed the existence of a God who, being good by definition, would never fool us into falsity.[2] The soul was immortal and immaterial, a 'thinking thing' that thinks it thinks it thinks, while the mortal, brute body, brain included, was an 'extended thing' Descartes likened to an automaton activated by pulleys. His was a tight system, within which animals – dogs included – could not be allowed immortal souls.

It is true that our awareness of being aware – our 'meta-cognitive' capacity, as it has usefully been called over the past fifty years – is what seems to define us as humans, a species

8

set apart from the rest of the animal realm.[3] It manifests in meaningful symbolic form – the arts, religions, ideas, sciences and technologies – that no other creature can create, not in such a sophisticated form at any rate. Like some other animals, we make meaning and social communities out of abstract signs and symbols, such as language. But unlike other animals we use language and other symbols to represent and contemplate ourselves and others, emotions and concepts, events and facts, past, present and future. We create stories and representations, and we remember them, inscribing ourselves and our lives through time, in order to confer meaning on our lives – of whose finiteness we are so terribly conscious. The dualist position has been tenacious throughout the history of thought, and it remains so, for it seems intuitively right: how could my complex thoughts have anything to do with matter? We hold on to our exceptional status within the created realm – our speciesism – no matter how destructive of our natural environment it has proved to be. Our impressive metacognitive capacity and our precious sense of meaning may seem to us to transcend our biology.

Yet these would not exist without our bodies. As we have known since Darwin, we are evolved animals, and we are born, and die, as feeling, sensorial, breathing, potentially endangered, usually resilient, time-bound bodies connected to other beings. When Descartes so imaginatively sundered mind and body, thereby ensuring the consoling immortality of a lone immaterial human soul ensconced within our imperfect, often ailing mortal frame (in part to reassure Church authorities), he also deprived beasts of all cognition and sensation, turning them into mere equivalents of automata.[4] Dog lovers at the time were none too happy. And in fact his strong mind–body dualism, as it is known, was criticized by many from the very start, with some of his contemporaries asking how an immaterial thought and a material mind could interact at all – how the thought of lifting my arm would trigger the movement, or how a blow to that arm would cause the feeling of pain. I now realize that my mother's apron was not just a quotation, but a spoof. 'Take that, René,' the dog seemed to say.

Descartes did imagine a locus of the mind–brain interaction – in the pineal gland, because of its central location between the two brain hemispheres. To be fair, he could tell as well as anyone that damage to the brain results in damage to mental life. He also accepted that emotions were at once corporeal and mental.[5] And there were always strong, alternative theories to his division of mind from body, such as those of vitalists, who argued for the inherence of soul in body.[6] Many physicians, attuned to the realities of ailing patients, adopted Gassendism, based on an adaptation by French philosopher Pierre Gassendi of ancient atomism to Christianity, and held on tight to the notion first developed in the fifth century BC by Aristotle that humans were on a continuum with the rest of creation. The philosopher Margaret Cavendish developed this view: 'neither can I perceive that man is a monopolist of all reason, or animals of all sense, but that sense and reason are in other creatures as well as in man and animals', she wrote.[7] There were attempts at a psychosomatic medicine, in line with the humoural, holistic model of psychology and medicine that had also prevailed since the ancient Greeks – and about which I wrote a book.[8] Spinoza, in reaction to Descartes, reconceived Nature and God as one substance. But despite alternative currents of thought, Descartes's dualism held strong for a long time, in various guises and many places. Over the eighteenth century, it gradually became absorbed into medicine, which turned the body into a machine-like mechanism. And modern mainstream medicine still chops us up into discrete bits.

Over the course of the eighteenth and nineteenth centuries, as materialism rose along with secularism, the notion of a separate, immaterial soul lost its function. Gradually, the empirical study of the mind became enmeshed with the philosophical study of knowledge and self. Psychology became scientific over the second half of the nineteenth century, and started encompassing questions that until then had been exclusively the domain of philosophy, such as perception, attention, imagination, emotion, the will and consciousness. This happened in particular under the impetus of the German physiologist and philosopher Wilhelm Wundt, who coined the notion of a 'scientific psychology', Théodule Ribot in France[9] and, most notably, William James in the US, whose *The Principles of Psychology* was first published in 1890 in New York and is still read today. In parallel, modern neurology and psychiatry were taking shape alongside accelerating knowledge of the anatomy and physiology of the brain and nervous system.[10] This meeting of scientific psychology with modern anatomical findings has led to the mind sciences of today. It has also meant that for many people it has become a given that our capacities are on a continuum with those of other animals, and that matter itself is complex enough that we do not need immortal, immaterial souls to explore our own ability to think, feel and have consciousness. We have, for the most part, accepted that we cannot escape our mortal frame.[11]

But this shift back to our embodied nature remains fraught. In the 1920s, behavioural psychologists had extended the Cartesian model by positing that behaviour was just the outcome of reflex-like responses to environmental stimuli, rather than manifestations of emotionally rich intentions.[12] From the 1950s on, the cognitive sciences outgrew the behaviourist model, absorbing neuroscience and evolutionary theory into their accounts of individual and social psychology, and elaborating scientific protocols that put the mind back behind the behaviour. For a while, the belief prevailed in these cognitive sciences that our brain was a machine that computed information, performing algorithmic functions that could be studied irrespective of the biological structures upon which they operated – as if biology were incidental to the higher activities of a brain separate from the body. The old mind–body dualism had given way to a brain–body dualism, one that persists in many scientific corners.[13]

At the same time, knowledge of the brain, oft dubbed the most complex object in the universe, has been growing tremendously over the past thirty years – in part with the help of artificial intelligence. We don't yet know nearly enough to counter the ravages of the neurodegeneration that is affecting my mother, as well as millions of others. But technological advances in brain imaging, in particular, are allowing for an increasingly sophisticated understanding of the brain in terms of interconnected networks. Neurophysiology, genetics, molecular biology, biochemistry and biophysics are together yielding a better understanding of neurons and neurotransmitters. Yet, the biological neurosciences generate hypotheses about the generic brain, deal with models, statistics, averages, and study cohorts.[14] And so they can be prone to ignoring two essential, and related, components of the experiencing mind: the complex, potentially ailing, individual body in which the brain is ensconced, and the embeddedness of this embodied brain in the social world.[15]

Attention to the body, however, has also intensified over the past two decades, within both the sciences and the humanities. Empirical approaches to the big questions have been converging productively with philosophical ones, leading to the acknowledgement that the emotions generated in the body are central to cognition and communication, and to producing insights into perception and sensation, the sense of time, as well as the sense of agency (that is, the sense of being the initiator of an action), the related sense of body-ownership (that is, the sense that the body and its actions are one's own) and, in general terms, the embodied sense of self. An increasingly detailed picture is also emerging of the relation of cerebral activity to our other vital organs – in particular the heart and the gut – and of the mechanisms of 'interoception', that is, the experience of our body from within, and the perception of bodily sensations whether we attend to them or not. The biologically real, relational, feeling body that is embedded in the world has re-entered the mind, informing how we understand the self as an inherently social entity, and also how it can diverge from the body's reality[16] – that is, how, in illness, we do not always feel ourselves to be what we are.[17]

What I call this 'interoceptive turn' is momentous, in that it may enable us to understand ourselves in scientific terms better than has ever been possible before.[18] The brain serves the body, not the other way round, as the neuroscientist Antonio Damasio has put it. It was Damasio who initiated the neuroscientific break from brain–body dualism in 1994, with the publication of his epochal first book, *Descartes's Error*, which showed how embodied emotional processes are integrated into rational ones.[19] Since then, the study of the corporeal, feeling and emotional self has been growing richer by the day, and studies of interoception and the embodied sense of self have been growing exponentially. This shift has helped undermine the view of the brain as an information-processing machine that can be understood apart from the rest of the body, as if we were not fully biological creatures. It is grounding what we may intuitively feel about ourselves in scientific detail and yielding tremendous insight into what it is that may be breaking down when the always-embodied sense of self is disrupted, when we cease to feel our body as our own. In conjunction with developmental psychology and psychoanalysis, it also shows how the embodied sense of self is always shaped in relation to others, from our first carers in infancy to the people with whom we share our lives, and to the societies in which we live.[20]

For the mind is inherently relational, not isolated. It includes a nervous system that develops in relation to other people. From birth on and even before – from the very beginning of fetal development – we live with, and in communication with, each other. Indeed, we have evolved in such a way that our cognitive and emotive functions are embedded within the need to communicate, cooperate, compete – to explore and exploit.[21] We need others to survive, and to endow a life with meaning. Cognitive and emotional disturbances are, crucially, disturbances in our capacity to be in the world and to be with *others*. The question remains, then, how these insights can pan out clinically: when, in trying to care for people whose minds have veered off course, neurologists and psychiatrists must focus on an *individual's* specific functions and dysfunctions in all their complexity.[22]

It is to answer this question that, for about eighteen months, I became a fly on the wall at the weekly clinical meetings of a neuropsychiatry unit at the Pitié-Salpêtrière hospital. Here the individual patient, not the theory, was centre stage. The person, not the model, was under scrutiny. This book recounts a selection of those meetings, which I had the chance to attend on the invitation of an old acquaintance, a neurologist who investigates consciousness at the same hospital. (At the time of writing, the unit has interrupted these weekly meetings, which had been going on for about seven years.) Some of the patients were severely ill. But most could have been you or me: they walked in as anonymous, ordinary-looking individuals, and became patients only upon entering the hospital room. They chose to consult that unit in particular, or were sent in by family or other doctors, because their disturbances had an unclear cause or diagnosis, and called for in-depth investigation. I was privy to their exceptionally lengthy examinations. I heard their medical histories, and witnessed tales of fragility, loss, confusion, resilience, and sometimes of healing, all rooted within complex familial and social circumstances. There was – is – no end to the variety of stories lived and told.

Selecting those that are most revealing of the entwinement of brain and body, I tell some of these stories here. All names have been changed and details altered to preserve anonymity. But the stories here are all based on what I heard. Unlike my mother's, they are fragments of lives of which I knew nothing beyond what was presented on the day: I saw each patient only once and heard all the information I convey here during that single consultation. Yet all of them, I realized as I delved deeper into the neurosciences, tell us something about what it takes to construct a self, what it means to lose oneself, and how one can find oneself again. Each one is a testimony to the fascinating complexity of each human life, and each human mind.

These are not professional clinical accounts; they are not remotely supposed to be usable medically. I sat with the doctors once the patients had left, as neither doctor nor patient (though all of us are potential patients). Nor am I a scientist, and this is not a book about the brain any more than it is a handbook of neurology or psychiatry. People who have read books by Oliver Sacks may expect familiar territory. But though he too told the stories of patients – and he did so with a novelist's skill – he was a practising neurologist, while I have no formal scientific or clinical training. Rather I am exploring as a philosopher how to connect person, patient and brain, with the tools of science and on the basis of the latest research. My perspective is also, by now, that of a daughter mourning the strangely progressive loss of her mother – I could be one of the relatives who sometimes accompanied the patient to that consulting room, close witnesses who held on to the threads as they were unspooling.

But while I attended the sessions, mourning had not yet begun. I simply witnessed knowledge in action, as well as the gaps around the knowledge, what we cannot know about the life lived – the sensations felt by the people who undergo testing, answer questions and expose themselves in order to be helped. I call myself a 'science humanist': I am interested in drawing connections, apparent or hidden. Between the meaningful, felt stories we tell ourselves – those that clinicians use in their clinical practice – and what the scientific studies and the always provisional theories these yield tell about us. Between seen behaviour and mapped nervous system. Between the state of health and the state of illness. And between mind and brain, brain and body, body and world, world and selves.

These connections need to be drawn between categories of knowledge and disciplines that have been imposed upon one dimension, within which there are many gradations.[23] Theoretical neuroscience and psychology can tell us a lot about our thinking and feeling selves, but most people don't use such scientific knowledge in daily life. It constitutes a basis for this book but remains mostly 'backstage'. You will find plenty of references in the endnotes, which develop some of the scientific, historical and philosophical ideas mentioned in the text and provide sources for those who want to know more. It seems important to bring to light this high-end scientific research, which is usually confined to academic circles, and to put it to work throughout these pages –– to transfer it to the phenomenology of a lived life. Indeed, much as our illnesses can reveal a lot about our deepest nature, neurologists and psychiatrists faced with confused or distressed patients cannot make much use of sophisticated theoretical analyses, even when they also engage in translational – that is, clinically applicable – research.

This is in part because, while each patient presents with a case of something, no one case is ever the same as another, and because pathology and normality are on a continuum.[24] A clinician treats a person, not a disease. And each person is a unique configuration of features we all share: one cannot integrate this individuality in diagnostic or treatment protocol. Both science and medicine rely on statistical generalizability. They produce models and charts to which we can never reduce lives, values and stories. The scientist's job is to study a condition that may signal a disease. The doctor's job is to treat the one patient, though in order to do so, he or she must also square the unique individual with the generalizable case – but your story will always differ from mine.

I had always felt that the science and the philosophy I had been reading and writing about for twenty odd years enriched my intuitions – born of introspection not unlike that of the dog on the apron – about the ways in which thought and emotions constantly inform each other, and about the processes of my own introspective mind.[25] This book emerges out of my wish to expand my area of enquiry beyond my comfort zone. I wanted to understand how the felt experience of individuals in need of clinical attention can enrich, and be enriched by, the constantly evolving scientific knowledge that generally permeates our culture and informs medical care – in ways both positive and negative. I wanted, further, to explore how specific scientific accounts of the embodied mind can bear on the experience of being conscious, flawed, uncertain – teetering as we all are on the cliff edge that is our state of health.

But I had no inkling when I first sat down at the meetings at the Pitié-Salpêtrière how poignant, humbling, and transformative they would prove to be. Nor that they would help prepare me to face the neurological illness of my own mother. Or that I would be reckoning one day with the gap between the story told and the story lived. Between the writer and the reader. Between then and the evanescent now. It is my hope that these pages will help you too – to understand yourself, and those around you, in illness and in health.

2

The Old Campus

Sometimes the breakdown does lead to a kind of cure, and the word 'health' turns up again.

Donald W. Winnicott,
'The Concept of a Healthy Individual' (1967),
in *Home is Where We Start From*

One enters the Pitié-Salpêtrière grounds through arches set within an august seventeenth-century façade – a classified monument. Behind stands a well-proportioned church from the same era. It is a beautiful place, a town within the city, with its own street names, quarters, and gardens. A grassy common at its centre – a rare occurrence in Paris – is popular with staff and medical students for lunchtime picnics when weather permits, and otherwise is open to anyone who happens to stroll in. There is rarely anything joyful in having to go to hospital; if one does, one usually hopes to be able to leave it as soon as possible. But a hospital is also a vibrant, creative workplace dedicated to the care of others. And I loved my weekly visits to the Pitié-Salpêtrière. I loved the classical architecture, the tasteful and well-tended flowerbeds that dot the campus, the buzzing, multifarious activity. I even loved going there with my mother when she visited her neurologist.

The first time I took her for her consultation with him, I was still attending the sessions at which the same man examined the patients with his colleagues, just a few buildings away. But now my own mother was his patient, and I could observe his empathy and the refined clinical skills I had seen him use with other patients as he interacted with her. I was then on the other side of the table, next to her. No longer a witness to the travails of an unknown patient. Yet my observing, detached self remained. I tried to see what he saw. And at each subsequent visit, as her lucidity was progressively fading, I felt increasingly grateful for the knowledge I had been able to glean from the sessions he had welcomed me to.

Here we were, then. We knew what this was. No need to check, no need to test. We saw the signs. I was the daughter, not the doctor, but still, by that point I was well prepared. We exchanged some observations, I used the vocabulary I had learned. We also knew what lay ahead. But besides attaching technical words to the cerebral dysfunctions, there was nothing he could do. Not even one of the most thoughtful neurologists in one of the best neurology departments anywhere can stop the process we know as dementia.

One of the largest hospitals in Europe, the Pitié-Salpêtrière is particularly well known for its neurology and psychiatry departments, not only because of their high calibre and exceptional staff, but also because they have a long, rich history. This history calls for a brief retelling here, all the more so because it relates directly to the concerns of this book. For a long time, it was just La Salpêtrière, a home for indigents of all sorts – prostitutes and the insane – that was also a sinister detention centre and an elderly women's hospice. It had been founded by King Louis XIV on the grounds of a saltpetre factory which gave its name to the hospice. By the time the Revolution broke out in 1789, it housed some 8,000 indigents, all female, within a space that was intended to hold 4,000 at most. It was the largest hospice in the world.[1] But things started changing in 1795, at the tail end of the Revolution, when a doctor named Philippe Pinel became chief physician at La Salpêtrière. He had developed an expertise in mental illness and had worked at the then notoriously sinister Bicêtre hospice for men just outside Paris as chief physician, caring for what we today call psychiatric patients.

The term psychiatry was actually only first coined in the early nineteenth century, and did not become current for several decades.[2] In the late 1700s, mentally ill patients were still considered incurable: they were called 'aliénés', held in shackles in airless, dark and dank, insalubrious prisons, alongside prostitutes and criminals. Pinel was a force for change, and he is remembered for instituting the humane treatment of these patients. He was in fact inspired in this by an empathic superintendent at Bicêtre who removed the shackles of the inmates there and spent time observing and listening to them. Pinel famously proceeded to do the same when he arrived at La Salpêtrière, unshackling the patients and observing them over time. And he wrote a hugely influential classification of diseases – a nosology - in which mental disorders formed an important, precisely calibrated subgroup.[3]

A protégé of Pinel was Jean-Etienne-Dominique Esquirol, who joined the Salpêtrière soon after Pinel, and started in 1817 to teach there the first courses in psychiatry in the country. Both men believed in the importance of drawing up detailed case histories to understand mental illness. Both emphasized the power of a psychologically informed approach to initiating the cure of patients, regarding them as socially situated persons in thrall to passions and in need of help. Esquirol believed that rational faculties remained present even when they weren't conscious, to the extent that by attending to them the doctor could make inroads into the patient's mind.[4] He also emphasized the impact of social conditions on mental health, touring asylums for the insane nationwide and reporting officially on their (ghastly) conditions.[5] This was a time when physicians who were heirs at once to Enlightenment materialism and to Revolutionary ideals of justice were becoming aware of the social dimension of health: mental illness was now seen as a product of social and medical circumstance, and therefore was curable, rather than a lifelong condemnation and a 'moral' blight. It is within this progressive context that modern neuropsychiatry started taking shape.[6] And La Salpêtrière became over the course of the nineteenth century an international centre at the cutting edge of research into the sciences of the mind, with its own school.[7]

The reputation of the hospice grew especially during the tenure of Jean Martin Charcot, one of its most celebrated alumni. Over three previous decades, starting in 1862, he had dealt with various branches of medicine, but he focused on the field of neurology, and in 1882 founded at La Salpêtrière the first ever European clinic of neurology. We owe to him the identification of many neurological diseases and syndromes, in particular multiple sclerosis, and the terrible amyotrophic lateral sclerosis, or ALS, which remains known as 'Charcot's disease', or Lou Gehrig's disease in the United States. Crucially for the development of neurology and neuroscience, he developed the so-called 'anatomo-clinical' method of correlating clinical symptoms with cerebral lesions observed post-mortem, thereby helping to establish that the brain was constituted of specialized areas associated with specific functions, rather than being a homogeneous mass.[8] He also, notably, made use of the then novel technologies of photography and electrophysiology.[9]

But Charcot's name is also associated with his important studies of hysteria and the theatrical settings of his demonstrations, criticized even at the time.[10] The study of hysteria has its own long history. The term refers etymologically to the Greek *hystera* for womb, and in ancient medicine it denoted ailments connected with a 'wandering womb'. It was the so-called female malady, though by the seventeenth and eighteenth centuries, it had a male equivalent in so-called hypochondria. Both terms named a mental disorder made manifest in the body – that is, somatized.[11] In Charcot's day, La Salpêtrière was still a refuge for distressed women.[12] A few of these traumatized women who displayed real enough hysterical symptoms became Charcot's patients. He also opened a ward for men – they too were from the working classes, since those from the middle and upper classes could afford private doctors and more salubrious clinics. And he conducted his studies on both men and women, in a departure from what he had learned earlier as an intern for physician Pierre-Adolphe Piorry, who still believed hysteria was a female malady.[13] Charcot thought of what he called hysteria as a specific, organic, neurological disease that could be studied as such even though no neurological lesions were visible on autopsies of hysteric patients.[14] Unlike the epileptics in his charge, hysterics, he found, could be uniquely hypnotized – it was hypnosis that enabled the study of hysteria: in the course of hypnosis they underwent an 'artificial' hysteria during which the trauma that had presumably caused the pathology was re-enacted.

What to some extent undermined the public perception of Charcot's legacy is that he 'displayed', and had photographed, young women undergoing these hypnosis-induced hysterical seizures in an elaborate theatricality, which he divided into four stages. As Lisa Appignanesi writes in her account of this episode:

So widely diffused were the dramatic images recording the four stages of the hysterical attack, so much talked about were Charcot's hysterics, it is hardly surprising that various forms of contemporary malaise found their way into an unconscious mimicking of the popularized symptoms.[15]

His famous Tuesday lessons were open to the public. Students, most of them male (there were not many female medical students, though he encouraged them), alongside writers and artists, flocked to watch, observe, learn. But there was also a voyeuristic element to his displays of female suffering that later contributed to his dismissal as a result of claims by some of his colleagues that he was a charlatan. A famous canvas painted in 1887 of a Charcot Tuesday lesson shows one of the most well known of the 'grandes hystériques', the unfortunate Blanche Wittmann, held in the arms of Charcot's favourite student, Joseph Babinski, while Charcot demonstrates hypnosis. It must be remembered, however, that Charcot was an early promoter of women in medicine.[16]

A young neurology student, Sigmund Freud, was amongst the Charcot enthusiasts when he was in Paris in 1885, and in 1886 he even translated Charcot into German upon his return to Vienna. But a debate pitted Charcot against a neurologist called Hippolyte Bernheim who dismissed hypnosis as 'psycho-genic suggestion' – symptoms provoked under the therapist's influence – and this debate was instrumental in paving the way to Freud's distancing himself from Charcot's circle and claims, and the shift, from 1888, to the method he eventually developed into psychoanalysis.[17] Back in Vienna, he found a new mentor in the physician Joseph Breuer, who had been working with patient 'Anna O', treating her symptoms of hysteria through what she herself named the *talking* cure'.[18] For his part, in Paris, Babinski became a renowned clinical neurologist (known especially for his work on reflexes), who also distinguished 'organic' diseases from psychiatric ones, determining that hysteria belonged to the latter group. The division endures today between neurological disorders deemed to be endowed with an organic basis, and psychiatric ones deemed not to be.

Much of the history of this division between structural and functional – between a precise, potentially visible injury within the central nervous system and a diffuse ailment involving mental states but not readily identifiable with a precise injury

– was played out on the Salpêtrière grounds. Psychiatry and neurology were not yet separate fields at the time of Charcot, the young Freud, and others. A person like my mother, afflicted with dementia, would belong to the same category of patient as someone afflicted with what the German psychiatrist Emil Kraepelin first named schizophrenia. He was a colleague of Aloïs Alzheimer, who discovered, and after whom was named, the dementia probably afflicting my mother.[19] The mind-brain was one entity, and its disturbances required attention to the whole person – to the sensorimotor dimension as well as to general mood, to the nervous system as well as to the more vague category of affect, which encompasses the experience of feelings, such as emotions or moods.

Over the course of the twentieth century, the domains diverged. Neurology focused on symptoms related to organic, cerebral changes, while psychiatry concerned itself with behavioral disturbances of a functional nature – that is, with no clear organic basis. The one is close to internal medicine. The other, which was often connected to psychoanalysis, is concerned with the individual psyche. But by now the distinction is vexed, culturally conditioned, and begs as many questions as the parallel distinction between brain and mind. The assignation of a disorder to an area of enquiry is biased in a way that is similar to that of naming it. We assume that there are distinct categories into which the disorders of the mind fit, as if health and illness did not belong to a dimensional continuum, and in the absence of a complete understanding of what the mind is and how it works.[20] This separation also creates a clinical culture that may not always help patients, insofar as it reflects and perpetuates the old division of mind and body. And as we will see throughout this book, the very rationale of this old division is disappearing.[21]

The mental asylum at the La Salpêtrière hospice remained open for a while longer, until 1921. The hospice only became a hospital in 1968. By that point it had been renamed Hôpital Pitié-Salpêtrière (following its merger with an early seventeenth-century hospital called Pitié that had moved in 1911 to an adjacent lot), and it began to grow in size and reputation. Today buildings and streets there bear the names of celebrated doctors from the more or less distant past, while some of the buildings devoted to diseases of the nervous system are named after more recent neurologists. There is a rue Esquirol, a Pinel building, a large Babinski building, and the lecture theatre is named after Charcot.

It seems fitting that the meetings of the neuropsychiatry unit I attended took place just around the corner from the lecture theatre. For the very idea of this unit can be seen as another episode in the history of the division of psychiatry from neurology. Its purpose was to welcome patients whose symptoms related to both, and whose diagnosis was all the more fraught given that neuropsychiatry ceased to be a clinical speciality in France in the late 1960s. The unit met in a very bright top-floor room overlooking the modern buildings that lie to the south of the hospital. Floor-to-ceiling windows lined one side of the small room. There was a large table in the middle and a whiteboard at one end, some chairs and stools. Never more than a dozen people present. Senior neurologists and a senior psychiatrist, junior residents, interns, students – all clad in hospital whites. Sometimes an outsider like myself, sometimes a colleague from another clinic – not in whites. The proceedings were typical of those of any clinical meeting and started with the presentation of the medical history, inter-rupted by comments, questions, clarifications. But what was not typical was the lengthy examination of the patient that fol-lowed – sometimes for up to an hour. Discussions of cases, following the examination, never more than three per session and usually just two, could last a long time as well. In that respect, this particular meeting was exceptional: time is a precious commodity in the medical world. What was also exceptional was the – still all too rare – dialogue between neurologists and psychiatrists.

The openness of these sessions to an outsider like myself was unusual. I did feel sometimes I was peering into a sacred inner sanctum, witness to something at once private and universal – the uniqueness and commonality of suffering. But this was no Charcot Tuesday. These meetings were discreet. There was no display, nothing programmatic, and certainly nothing voyeuristic there. Granted, it may seem odd to sit in on a medical consultation; it would indeed be hard to imagine allowing external visitors to observe a consultation with a dermatologist, or a gastro-enterologist – and it would be of limited, specialized interest to do so. Nor would anyone think of listening in on a psychotherapy session. If it was possible for me to sit in on the neuropsychiatry clinics, it was because there was no intimacy, no undressing, no poking about beneath the skin. Observing where a person has ceased to know herself fully, the brain hitting against its blank spots, the space of self and consciousness transformed – that is closer to putting neuro-science in practice. It is even philosophically provocative. I was welcomed in because matters of mind matter so centrally to us all.

3

The Lost Years

We are all a hotchpotch of parts, so diverse and so loosely held together that each one, at every moment, pulls its own way. And there is as much difference between us and ourselves, as there is between us and others.

Michel de Montaigne,
'On the inconstancy of our actions',
in *Essays*, vol. II (1588)

A young woman lost her memory: I had already decided to tell her story before all the others when my mother read the chapter on her last ever Eurostar trip, in late 2018. We were on our way to London to attend a Christmas party at my sister's. We have taken many Eurostar trips together, ever since the train was inaugurated in 1995. When I ask her if she remembers, sometimes she responds, chuckling and smiling, 'of course I remember!' But there is no way of knowing what this remembering refers to. When she read an early draft of this chapter, which was still not thought through, I don't think she really understood much. She said it was 'very interesting'. On the first night of our stay at Alba's house in London, she asked me where we were going to sleep, anxiously pointing at her suitcase, and saying, 'I have to go home now.' I was dismayed: this was a first. A harbinger of what was to come. Later, she woke up at 2.00 a.m. and got dressed and made up, ready to go out. When we arrived back in Paris two days later, she asserted, as the Eurostar slowed down at the Gare du Nord, that we had arrived in London. An old woman was losing her memory. Was she losing herself, too? There is a gradation to loss. Her general confusion was intermittent, but it was gradually becoming a particular pathology.

The course of such an illness must be recorded in detail to make any medical sense. A patient's medical history is parallel to a life history and, unless or until it takes over all of life, it only overlaps with it intermittently. The medical history is called 'anamnesis' – and this is what the doctors called it in the hospital room. Anamnesis is an ancient Greek word that originally denoted a recollection of past lives, a memory from a past incarnation – 'mimnisko', from which anamnesis is formed, means to 'call to mind'. Plato referred centrally to anamnesis in his dialogues *Phaedo* and *Meno* when puzzling out how one can come to know something one has never encountered. How can we know what we are looking for if we have never seen it, he wondered? Socrates, as always, had an answer: if we do know what we are looking for, then we already know what it is. And so it must be that we forget with each new incarnation what the soul already knows and re-learns with each life. So, according to Plato's Socrates, learning is just remembering.[1] It seems remarkable that this very term of anamnesis should be used in modern times to denote a medical history, encapsulating what turns a person into a patient, what creates the separation between the individual coming in for a clinical examination, and the white-clad, presumably healthy, thoughtful people discussing that person around a table. Lurking within this association is a sense – if one takes literally the ancient Greek meaning of anamnesis – that to tell a medical history is also to retrieve some of the forgotten truths of a person's life.

◆

It is admittedly unclear what truths were conveyed by the anamnesis of the patient I saw one autumn morning during the first weeks of my attending the neuropsychiatry unit. She was a thirty-eight-year-old woman, with a pleasant, bespectacled face. I shall call her Vanessa. As was the case for all the patients chosen for discussion by the members of the unit, her thick file was waiting in the middle of the table, her last name inscribed on its spine in black marker. Hers was a strange, mysterious story. She had told it many times to various doctors in other medical services since an accident that had occurred just two years before. The junior doctor read this compendium of notes and accounts from a computer screen, as was the protocol for each session, which always began with the anamnesis.

One day two years ago, the junior doctor read out before she entered the room, Vanessa fainted and fell into a hyperglycemic coma because of undiagnosed diabetes. When she came to in the hospital room, she had no idea where she was. She didn't recognize the man sitting at her bedside as her husband. She underwent a series of tests, including brain scans, one of which was an MRI that showed a small atrophy of the internal temporal hippocampus. The hippocampus is essential in the processing of memory. The episode, doctors soon realized, had given way to massive amnesia, a type called 'retrograde' amnesia: when she awoke, she had in fact forgotten a whole swathe of the life that had preceded her coma.[2] Ten whole years of her life were gone.

The scale of what such a loss signifies emerged when she arrived in the small room at the hospital, took a seat, and, prompted by one of the neurologists, started describing what she had experienced. She told us that she hadn't recognized the countryside home she returned to after being released from hospital but recalled still living alone in a flat in the city, as a student. She also thought she was single, certainly not married to that particular man. She had considered herself to be quite slim, but now felt alarmingly fat (she was indeed very overweight). She did not recognize her life, and her tastes and ideas had changed. On this other side of the coma, she believed herself to be twenty-eight rather than her actual age of thirty-eight. In her mind the political scene was as it had been in 2006. Even her speech mannerisms dated to then, the doctors had noted on her anamnesis. It was as if she had rewound time. She knew who she was, she assured us, but she felt lost. Calm, but lost. With the help of family and friends, as well as the man who was her husband, she managed to retrieve some information about the lost years, bit by bit, although, she said, it felt external to her. This was why she was consulting the doctors at the Pitié-Salpêtrière again, the same ones who had seen her after the accident had first happened, desperate to continue taking hold of her life, to trace some sort of line between this odd present and what she knew she was. All the more so since she had been known to have an exceptional memory: people were always impressed with her capacity for flawless recall, she told us. She had been a policy advisor but felt unable to return to work after the accident, because she couldn't recognize colleagues and clients who greeted her and knew her from before, referring to events that had disappeared into the chasm. She complained of being tired and having difficulty in concentrating, which made it hard for her to read. She was now teaching a remedial writing class in a school. She had even registered as disabled. She wanted her health and life back.

Yet I noticed that beyond the lost decade, her memory seemed to function perfectly well. She struck me as on the ball, quick-witted and aware. In fact she seemed like a perfectly normal young woman. Vanessa was coherent as she spoke. She herself reported that somehow she had reconstructed herself. The amnesic blank had placed itself within her life narrative, had become an aspect of who she was by now. She told us that she succeeded in recognizing as a part of her past some of the elements her entourage kept giving her, even retrieving memories unprompted. Yet she also told us that none of these retrieved elements ever felt like her own, inalienable experience. She had knowledge that things had happened, that she had married a man with whom she was in love at the time, and had gone on a six-month honeymoon, for instance, but without it constituting intimate, self-referential knowledge. It did not *feel like* anything. She certainly could not remember ever having been in love with that blond husband who did not remotely look like her ideal, and from whom she was now divorcing. (She had always preferred dark types, anyway, she said.) The retrieved elements weren't part of a past she could own, or of her self-consciousness. They were merely familiar, and external to her feeling self: they partook, one would say in technical terms, of noetic or intellective, not autonoetic or self-aware consciousness.[3] She did not *feel* present within these memories even though she *knew* they were of events that she had lived. In other words – not her own words, but the theoretical terms used by the psychiatrist, and that helped interpret what she was saying – they were just a bit of semantic memory, which is the general knowledge we need to live day by day. They were no longer episodic memory: the long-term, autobiographical narration necessary to construct ourselves.[4]

We take our memory for granted until an aspect of it breaks down. This much is clear when dementia hits – as I have been finding out with my mother. When something goes wrong in its complex mechanism, we realize the extent to which experience is a meaningless vanishing point without it. Our self is the central experiencer that owns these memories, or to whom these memories refer. The self generates the memories that in turn define and constrain it, determining its path through time and how we understand, reconstruct our past and project ourselves into the future – however imaginary that path in fact may be. The sense of self, and of its embodied sensations, is at least in part tied into memory. It is constructed out of a continuously renewed, selective, unstable, yet apparently seamless remembering, a perpetual act of reconstruction that preserves the stability of the self. What we remember is also what we once *felt*: emotional memories are embodied memories, the output of interoceptive processes. But remembering is also to reconstruct the past within the present, and according to the present state of the embodied, feeling self. It is not the retrieval of a file from a container: it is a continual, dynamic process. Memories change as we remember. And crucially, this act of reconstruction also involves selective forgetting.[5]

Vanessa's stated anamnesis, in fact, did not seem to be her full story – precisely because it was a story about a story's missing elements. The neurologist examining her became more sceptical of what she was telling us as the examination proceeded. He started prompting her about her inability to return to her previous activities. He told her that maybe she suffered more from wanting to retrieve her memory than from the actual effects of the ten-year gap. Taking a broadly psychological view of her troubles, he offered that it was the fact of not remembering that perturbed her, given how much importance she had always attached to her flawless memory: it was a quality that had become part of her self-description, an identity card to herself and others. He believed she was suffering more from her old reliance on this quality, and the expectations it had created, than from the amnesia itself. She disagreed: 'to know where one is going,' she countered, 'one needs to know where one comes from.' The doctor pushed on, trying to encourage her to move forward. 'You can't re-invent the future,' he said. 'Try to dissociate the amnesia from its consequences – for all we know, the neurological or psychological mechanism that has produced your amnesia, whatever it may be, has stopped. You may be on the other side of it.

Yet you are making yourself live in its shadow. It's blocking you.'

Vanessa did listen. She had sought out help, after all, and it was clear that she owed it to herself, and to the doctors, to welcome it. She had not thought of her predicament as anything she was imposing on herself, she said, and so the suggestion struck her in its novelty. And she had had other amnesic episodes after the first, massive one. One morning, she told us – and the story had been part of the anamnesis as well – she had walked into the sitting room, naked, where some friends had gathered. She had then woken up two days later, in her own bed, having been hospitalized during that time without her having any recollection of either the embarrassing episode or the hospitalization. Another time, while hallucinating, she had conversations with absent people, and slept for days thereafter. No one knew how she had self-administered her insulin during those absences, yet she had managed to. In medical terms, those were paroxystic episodes – that is, short-lived and intense, with a sudden onset and end. And in this instance at least, they were not fully explained. Vanessa said she was afraid such an event could re-occur, anywhere, any time, even at work. The neurologist suggested perhaps she was simply afraid of losing control. 'But I forget!' she countered. 'Memory is control,' replied the psychiatrist. 'And it is also about losing control,' added the neurologist: 'How do you explain this story?' 'No idea, I'm not a doctor,' she replied. The psychiatrist's subsequent response made everyone laugh, and Vanessa smile: 'But usually patients are better than doctors!'

How could one lose ten years within a few hours, anyway? Where was her personal time? How could she get herself back on its track, and get it back in synch with the rest of the world's time? The two years since the accident were a temporal chaos. Direction, inner and outer, was lost. Space was a mess. She was living in a place she would never have dreamed of living in, with a man she didn't particularly like. He was a mystery. So was she, in a way. She was not herself. Yet she was herself. Though a far fatter version of what she knew herself to be, and laden with diabetes, to boot. It was a wild confusion. She had found a way to cope, somehow, over the past two years, simply because she had to. But she was still living in an interim place.

After she had left the room, the doctors wondered: what were Vanessa's lost memories, exactly? Had she really forgotten everything about those ten years? There was an oddity in Vanessa's account, they observed: the absence of a 'Ribot gradient'. Théodule Ribot, as mentioned earlier, was a French psychologist, who wrote influential treatises about emotions, the unconscious, the will, and memory. And this 'gradient' corresponded to a phenomenon he had observed in numerous patients, enough times that he thought of it as a 'law': the more remote the memory from the time of the onset of the retrograde amnesia, the stronger the recollection. 'The progressive destruction of memory,' Ribot wrote, 'follows a logical order, a law. It advances progressively from the unstable to the stable.'[6] The most recent memories have fewer associations and are not consolidated. The oldest ones are sensorial and instinctive, as Ribot put it, and have become an aspect of self: amnesia 'follows the path of least resistance, that is, of least organization'. Ribot's Law indexes the potency of a memory to time. According to psychologist and memory specialist Daniel Schacter, the reason for this may be that 'some memories are subject to a long-term consolidation process that allows them to become more resistant to disruption over time.'[7] If one stuck to the letter of Ribot's Law, Vanessa should have been able progressively to recollect events between 2016 and 2006, especially up to four years prior to the accident. But she claimed instead that the ten years were all gone: she had no memory gradient. The doctors in the room thought of this as a unique case in the annals of neurology: somehow, something was wrong.

There are exceptions to Ribot's Law, I realized when I later looked up discussions of it. And more fundamentally, the law-like character of the phenomenon Ribot first observed is disputable.[8] Still, because Vanessa was presenting with such an unusually clear-cut ten-year blank, the neurologists and psychiatrists felt they needed to probe a little further. During their discussion, together they tried to tease out what exactly was 'blocking' Vanessa. She would have had strong motivations to forget the ten years and yank them out of her autobiography, the psychiatrist offered: a marriage that had gone sour, her obesity that caused the diabetes and that in turn had brought on the hyperglycemic coma and the subsequent episodes. Perhaps it was convenient, unconsciously, for her to wake up at the age of twenty-eight, he went on, for in so doing she had divested herself of a – metaphorically and literally – weighty past.[9] She was free to start again, and she could have returned to her old job if she wanted to, despite what she had told the doctors. She had needed to update her memory traces in light of her emotional state (all our memories are somehow inflected by associated emotional states). How she had done so was a mystery. At any rate, she had succeeded in doing this so well that now she was at a loss within her present.[10]

The profoundly disruptive experience of amnesia reveals how our memory is multi-dimensional, and not at all comparable to a digital storage system, despite the tendency to make this comparison ever since computers appeared.[11] One very different type of amnesia from the one suffered by Vanessa is Transient Global Amnesia, or TGA for short.[12] I witnessed my mother undergo a TGA once, in the late 1990s – long before dementia appeared – when I was visiting her from London where I lived at the time. All of a sudden, after breakfast, she looked at me wide-eyed: 'What are you doing here?' she asked. She had no recollection of my having arrived the night before, of our lively dinner, or breakfast, or the conversation we had just been having literally seconds before. Then, just as suddenly, she returned to where she had stopped, and continued talking as though nothing had happened. I asked her: 'Do you realize that you just asked me what I was doing here, that you forgot everything about my arrival?' She had no idea what I was talking about. The to and fro between these two parallel, mutually exclusive dimensions – multiverses of sorts – continued for about twenty-four hours. Then it dissipated, and never returned. As is usually the case with TGA, it remained a fascinatingly bizarre occurrence, a moment without consequence, simply an eccentric experience to ponder. Though at a distance of some years it seems, post-hoc, to have been a portent of the permanent retreat into another dimension that is the mark of my mother's dementia.

A TGA is very different from the kind of retrograde amnesia Vanessa presented with. And it also differs fundamentally from the anteretrograde type that can be spectacular enough to be the stuff of movies, and which consists of the inability to form new memories. The most famous case of this is that of HM – Henry Molaison – an American who suffered from epilepsy, and whose life changed radically on 1 September 1953. That day, in an attempt to cure him, neurosurgeon William Beecher Scoville removed his medial temporal lobes, including his hippocampus, a structure in the cortex that developed early on in our evolution and that is essential for episodic, or autobiographical memory and at least the initial storage of new information. He was twenty-seven when the surgery took place. The epilepsy became more controllable, insofar as it involved the hippocampus. But otherwise, the intervention was a disaster. The only new memories he could acquire thereafter pertained to the recollection of the immediate past – that is, short-term memory, which he was unable to transform into long-term memory – and to the procedural memory we use to acquire and preserve motor skills, such as the ability to play an instrument, ride a bicycle, and so on. His episodic memory of events, conversations, or people following the surgery was debilitatingly gone. It was, however, nearly intact for everything preceding it – though there was also a mild retrograde amnesia. His case would prove invaluable for advancing the comprehension of memory, a human tragedy in the service of science.[13]

In a 1996 TV documentary called *Without Memory*, the Japanese director Hirokazu Kore-eda painted a poignant portrait of the life of someone who also was afflicted by ante-retrograde amnesia and deprived of the ability to create new memories.[14] He focused on a young man, Hiroshi Sekine, who, following abdominal surgery and the disastrous medical decision subsequently to withdraw his vitamin intake, develops a neurological condition called Wernicke's Korsakoff Syndrome – due to vitamin B deficiency.[15] The hippocampal damage is irreversible. The film begins four years after the operation, shot over time in Sekine's home, the camera and crew witnessing and recording Sekine's wife and children adapting to their beloved's condition. Over and over again each day, Sekine realizes what has happened, descending into confusion, unable to recall moments beyond their fleetingness. Emotions and consciousness have no continuity. Early on in the film, after his wife tells him again that he has lost his memory – a repetition more frequent than the rising sun, and as predictable – Sekine says: 'If only I could build an awareness of my own condition, beginning in the morning and in the course of a day, then I could find a way to collect my thoughts, but the way I am trembling now must indicate that I've just realized my condition for the first time.'

One major difference between the spectacular, highly

dramatic cases of HM and Sekine and that of Vanessa was that Sekine became painfully aware over and over again of his condition, a *Groundhog Day* of realization, while being perpetually unable to hold on to that awareness. In contrast, Vanessa's memory was operational again. She had a decade's worth of unrecovered memories, and a sense of detachment from the recovered ones, but she was otherwise healthy. She was not in the least unaware that she had forgotten. Her capacity to live, learn, work and love normally was not, or did not seem to be dramatically affected by the ten-year lacuna she reported. Yet there were those strange paroxystic episodes, such as the one when she slept for two days. And she was suffering. The wipe-out had, tsunami-like, swept away everything that had happened over ten years: life, work, marriage, some semantic memory, even some procedural memory – she awoke unable to use her iPhone, as if she'd reverted to 2006, when it did not exist. At the time of the incident, she had felt neither sadness, nor distress, nor panic. But progressively that strange sense of detachment she felt from what had been her own life started causing her discomfort and anxiety. She seemed normal, and lived normally enough, but it was precisely the disjuncture between how she felt and how she knew she appeared to others that was confusing to her.

So was there anything neurologically wrong? The discussion of Vanessa's case lasted a while. The hippocampal lesion seemed to have resolved, observed the doctors, since she was capable of storing inputs into short-term memory that consolidated into long-term memory in a perfectly standard way. She herself observed that her old capacity for recall was running smoothly. She had no 'dysexecutive syndrome', they observed, that is, problems with executive function, which pertains to the highly evolved frontal lobes of the human brain. It is involved in analysing information and solving problems, processing perceptions, sensations, and, indeed, memories, making coherent plans, organizing thoughts, and controlling impulses so as to be able to complete a task. Disruptions in that function can cause major problems in daily life but Vanessa had no such problems. Nor was she suffering from *identity* amnesia, which would have involved different cerebral regions. The distinction is important: one can forget events about one's life, or about the lives of others close to us for that matter, without forgetting who we are. The sense of self is distinct from the memories that partake of it: the self develops along with memories, but not all memories feed into the sense of self.[16] Memory has many aspects, some of them segregated from others. The forgetting of events, episodes or facts, does not change the content of the so-called 'core' self, which is based within our very body, not in the information we garner during our lives.[17] We all forget some of the plethora of information we take in every day. And what we choose to remember defines our identity only insofar as we choose to remember it.

As the discussion went on, an element from the anamnesis that had not been considered previously came to the fore: according to the MRI taken at the time of the incident, there was another area of Vanesa's brain that seemed slightly affected, called the medial prefrontal cortex (mPFC for short). It is an area that has been associated with decision-making and memory consolidation. Our capacity to make decisions does suppose appropriate judgement, which relies on remembered events and on the emotions associated with these events.[18] Perhaps, suggested one of the neurologists, the slight lesion that had been visible in the mPFC accounted for Vanessa's continued incapacity to access her episodic memory and make use of it.[19] Whether this was the case or not, however, the lesion was likely to have resolved, given the brain's plasticity. Was Vanessa redefining her identity, her body image and embodied sense of self – how she represented her body to herself – by *choosing* to forget? The doctors did not suggest this in so many words, but they implied as much.

There is a phenomenon called hypermnesia that is the obverse of amnesia: it is the inability to forget, to prune memories. And it can be as debilitating as the amnesic loss of memories. The effects of near-total recall tell us something about how we define ourselves not only by the perceptions we register but also by those we do not, and how we partly constitute our selves by filtering out information, inputs, and sensations. The great Russian neuropsychologist Alexander Luria studied such a case of hypermnesia and wrote it up as his classic book, *The Mind of a Mnemonist*, exploring the story of patient 'S', Solomon Sherevesky, whose extreme synaesthesia and episodic memory became a serious impediment in his daily life.[20] As Reed Johnson wrote in a revealing *New Yorker* article about Sherevesky, 'Deriving meaning from the world requires us to relinquish some of its texture,' and S had too full an experience of texture for the present to make sense.[21] It occurred to me that Vanessa was struggling to redefine her life's meaning in light of the changed texture afforded by her altered memory.

The notion that we may somehow, non-consciously *choose* what to remember as well as what to forget, which underlies the psychoanalytic process that Freud first developed, is in fact tied into the interpretation of amnesia as a sort of hysteria. This was the view of Pierre Janet, an eminent psychologist who joined Charcot at La Salpêtrière in 1889, directing the Psychological Laboratory there. Later, in 1902, he succeeded in Théodule Ribot's chair of experimental psychology at the Collège de France. He was a major influence on Freud. And it was almost as if Janet's ghost had appeared during the discussion of Vanessa, there in that bright little room at the top of a modern building near the Charcot auditorium. Janet believed that hysteria was the manifestation of what he understood as 'dissociation' following a trauma: it often took the form of amnesia, and just as Charcot had first established, it was amenable to hypnotic therapy.[22] In the state of hypnosis, memories could return.

Bernheim and his colleagues had discredited the use of hypnosis as mere 'suggestion' that was not founded in a physiological event. After Charcot's death in 1893, Janet found himself alone in upholding that hypnosis did have a neurobiological basis, firm in his belief that the very project of a scientific psychology depended on refuting the role of suggestion in hypnotic treatment. If all was mere 'suggestion', the mind was no longer a possible subject of scientific study, because there would be no firm distinction between the scientist and the subject.[23] Continued opposition to hypnosis by the neurological establishment at La Salpêtrière eventually led to his departure from the hospital, though his views found resonance in the United States. (William James wrote about Janet's studies at length in *The Principles of Psychology*.[24]) But even as hypnosis lost its neurological respectability, Janet's observation of a state of dissociation following a shock, translated principally as an amnesia that served as a defense against the shock, wove its way both into psychoanalysis and into psychiatry.

The term used to replace hysteria in our day varies: it can be conversion disorder (CD), psychogenic disease, or functional neurological disorder (FND). It is somatic symptom disorder (SSD) in the *DSM 5*, the latest edition of the *Diagnostic and Statistical Manual of Mental Disorders*, the American reference book for psychiatrists, and bodily distress disorder (BDD) in the *ICD-11*, the *DSM*'s European counterpart. All these initials refer to a syndrome which remains very common, and which manifests in somatic symptoms that do not correspond to any known organic disease.[25] A history of emotional trauma can or may not be present. If it is, its recall and replay through hypnosis or psychotherapy can solve the syndrome – or may not. There is little agreement as to the nature of this syndrome.

As the doctors at Pitié-Salpêtrière considered Vanessa's case in 2018, however, it seemed that they were starting to believe her amnesia was a form of conversion disorder – that it was, in Janet's appellation, psychogenic – and this, regardless of the presence or not in her brain of any neurological lesions. A psychogenic disorder is a syndrome without any visible organic basis that is the expression of some form of disturbance, emotional or otherwise. It is also a disturbance in the sense of agency, a disruption of the self as central agent in an action, emotion, or sensation: in 'dissociation', it is the self that dissociates.[26] But what did this interpretation mean to the clinicians, exactly? And what would it mean for Vanessa?

Vanessa's case was bewildering. But it was also on a continuum with ordinary experience, for memory is never seamless for anyone. Any of us can be at a loss for a word or a name on occasion, which we experience as an interruption, a nuisance, a puzzling manifestation of a hidden mechanism. It happens to me fairly frequently. These 'word losses' – *manque du mot* in French – are hiccups in semantic memory. They are not pathological, unless and until they become systematic, as they have in the case of my mother, and signal the beginning of a neurodegenerative disease such as Alzheimer's, whose signature protein plaques often start accumulating in the hippocampus. It is a common experience to misremember – in fact it is an integral part of remembering. In an essay called 'Speak, Memory', Oliver Sacks vividly describes his memory of an unexploded bomb in the family backyard during the Blitz: he is sure he has seen it – but he later finds out from his brother that he was away at the time.[27] We can often be absolutely certain that a memory is real when it is in fact fabricated from, say, a photograph. Memory is labile, and deeply entwined with imagination.

There are biological accounts of how this works. When a

memory is first encoded, mainly within the hippocampus, it is consolidated, and turns into a long-term memory – which in turn can be updated by new input that modifies it when it is reactivated, and reconsolidated.[28] According to one theory, the original context in which factual information – of the sort, say, that Athens is the capital of Greece – is acquired separates from it, even though it would seem that the factual information endures within the hippocampus. And so such remembered factual information derives from the various traces accrued over time.[29] Reactivation of the memory never occurs in the same circumstances as those in which it was first encoded, so it is constantly updated and modified. It is a bit like Schrödinger's cat: the second its existence is acknowledged, it is transformed, even by the tiniest amount. In other words, the very act of remembering transforms the memory.[30] And with each evocation of an episode, the initial memory trace becomes more fragile, and more labile. Oliver Sacks's essay title is a direct reference to Nabokov's multilayered memoir *Speak, Memory*, where words create seemingly true worlds but are nonetheless at the beck and call of memory's imaginative, creative wanderings. Nabokov acknowledged explicitly that he recreated his life as he wrote his memoir.[31] Today one would call it autofiction. We select what seems emotionally salient, and we confer emotional or narrative salience on what we select. Our strongest memories are those we have re-remembered, recalled, refabricated enough times that they become like quotations of the initially remembered experience, or distant, representations of it.

How different from this ordinary experience, this perpetual re-writing of our lives, was Vanessa's experience of a missing decade in her life? Again, what had she lost, exactly? Had she perhaps gained something else, emotionally, by forgetting? The perpetually dynamic quality of memory is what enables us to live our lives meaningfully, to imagine the future and remember the past. And we don't need modern science to know this. In the third century, the Church Father Saint Augustine had observed in a celebrated passage on memory and time in his *Confessions* that the future 'does not yet exist' and the past 'no longer exists'. Time is not objective: it is an 'extension of the mind itself', which performs the functions of 'expectation, attention, and memory'. And so 'everything which happens leaves an impression on [the mind], and this impression remains after the thing itself has ceased to be. It is the impression that I measure, since it is still present, not the thing itself, which makes the impression as it passes and then moves into the past.'[32] We construct a continuity out of our experience, indeed out of our very existence, thanks to those impressions Augustine speaks of, processed within our memory and also within our imagination; and imagination is in some sense the capacity to recombine in a novel way encoded perceptions and memories. We have a full life insofar as we can remember, and hence imagine without immediate input, people, events, places, facts, reactions, tastes, sounds, emotions, sensations – even creating fictional characters, for instance. Thinking itself recruits the imagination. We would be empty without that multiple, twin faculty of memory and imagination that enables stuff to stick, as it were – and for these very words I am typing as a form of written memory, to constitute sentences, and meaningful sense (words that I imagine you, the imagined reader, will one day be reading).[33]

Augustine had no access to the neurological knowledge we have today, of course. But what we intuitively feel to be the case about ourselves does often tend to be biologically the case about ourselves. At any rate, Augustine's description of memory and the experience of time is extraordinarily insightful. Later, Thomas Aquinas and other scholastic thinkers of the Middle Ages – whose philosophical practice consisted of the careful analysis of concepts – argued that the act of remembering can be an act of imagination: memories were based on images, or *phantasia*, acquired through the senses.[34] It remains a helpful idea: Vanessa had perhaps reconstructed a new recombination, a new continuity, by choosing her memories, and re-imagining herself through forgetting. Imagination powerfully shapes perception – including the perception we have of our own, embodied, self. For that matter, it must have felt peculiar for Vanessa to feel thin as she had been aged twenty-eight, and yet be fat as she was now. There was a disjuncture between her current body shape and the one she represented to herself now, and this disjuncture may well have been central to her experience, though the doctors did not ask her about it.[35] What they knew, and what she knew too, in a way, was that she had somehow played a trick on time, via her embodied memory, just as time had played a trick on her. There is evidence showing that episodic memory in particular does seem to share neuronal circuitry with the process of thinking about the future, just as the scholastic psychologists intuited.[36] Think (or remember, or imagine) how a memory of a conversation, an encounter, or a person's face, can quickly transform into speculation, planning, wondering about the future, and so on. Conversely, an amnesia affecting episodic memory also affects the ability to imagine the immediate future, or a person not present – the ability, in other words, to have any of the *phantasia* posited by the scholastic psychologists. Perhaps Vanessa felt stuck in her life and in her capacity to imagine the future because of her amnesia – and so, perhaps the initial impression she gave of functioning quite normally belied a deficit that had not resolved. Or perhaps, on the contrary, she had forgotten the past out of a fear of the future. But why after a coma? Was there a scientific way of understanding what had happened? Was there a scientific fact of the matter here? In other words, those of the writer Siri Hustvedt:

How does the subjective first-person phenomenal experience of a handicap relate to objective third-person
neurophysiology? In hysteria, this dilemma is particularly
urgent because the illness appears to reside in the hyphen
between brain and mind, obfuscating what we call psyche
and what we call soma.[37]

◆

A scientific investigation begins with a hypothesis. If this
hypothesis is about the human mind, it often is the outcome
of a hunch, a feeling about ordinary intersubjective experience.
Modern scientific findings about the mind often (though not
always) confirm what we already have intuited from experience
or thought through conceptually – hence the phenomenological depth of Augustine, or the clarity of the scholastic
model of the mind. By now psychologists have developed a
wide array of empirical means to test the sorts of intuitions
and theories we have had about ourselves ever since we evolved
into beings endowed with metacognition. And neuroscientists
look at the cerebral instantiation of psychological events – what
may be happening in the brain as these occur. Over the past
few decades, it has become possible to gather and interpret
data from brain imaging with far more sophistication than was
the case in the early days of this technology, during the 1990s.
Along with advances in technology and heightened power and
interpretive subtlety of brain imaging, has come a change in
the kind of cerebral activity one can investigate. We can now
look at how fine-grained aspects of experience occur. But even
then, the experience – what we live, feel, respond to – is not
reducible to the biological events underpinning it. Rather, the
biological picture we grasp may simply reflect our phenomenal
experience: we can only read a map if we have a key. So for
instance we can decide to look for the biological bases for

episodic and semantic memory respectively, but we must understand what those types of memory are in the first place, and how they differ. We usually identify types of memory first by referring to everyday experience – psychological investigations often begin on the same intuitive site as philosophical ones. The next step is to model that experience – to devise a schema that would give us a scientific understanding of the operations underlying it.

But there was no perfect scientific model for Vanessa's story. It was hard to tease out clinically in part because the medical interpretations relied on assumptions about the connections of mind, body and pathology that in turn had a cultural and philosophical history. I was intrigued by the clinical consensus that Vanessa presented with no major biological anomaly which could count as a structural cause for her current state, that there was no plausible neurological explanation for her admittedly disturbing experience. The absence of a Ribot gradient was, for the doctors, a key to this interpretation. (Though as already stated, there are exceptions to the Ribot gradient.) Granted, said one neurologist, temporal epilepsy was a plausible consideration, given her paroxystic episodes preceded by acoustic hallucinations: 'Ten years of recurrent epilepsy could, just, result in a lacuna such as hers, blocking episodic memory.' During the calm periods, her memory would be encoding correctly, he surmised, while its fluctuations would explain why her biographical account was so hard to follow. He noted that an EEG performed at the time of the episode had come out normal, but that it was worth performing a new one.

Still, whether the proposed EEG to re-open the possibility of epilepsy as a factor turned out positive or not, her lost decade begged for a psychological investigation, all the doctors agreed. After all, Vanessa was able to absorb new information about her erased life, and again, she had no identity amnesia, that is, no dissociative identity disorder (DID), as it is now called in the *DSM 5*. She knew who she was, and she had knowledge of her memory loss. This looked rather like a psychogenic amnesia, which the *DSM 5* as well as the *ICD-11* call 'dissociative amnesia', and which harks back to Janet. The chief psychiatrist suggested, with a measure of irony, that Vanessa was displaying 'an organic expression of regret' – even though the organic element was unknown – and that there was an element of 'hysterical hippocampal flow', because her story was so tortuous. Yes, this could be a case of conversion disorder, he concluded. The neurologist who had examined her agreed.

Janet's ghost still seemed to be standing in the corner of the room, watching the debate of his day about the distinction between structural and functional, neurology and psychiatry playing itself out here too, on his old turf. The fact that Vanessa's memory was currently normal need not mean that there was nothing organically wrong with her – but the organic dimension remained unknown.[38] Something had gone askew in how she was processing her memories, her self-narration, and her sense of agency. There had to be an organic event accompanying this transformation of her life, I pondered, however complex the event, and however undetectable with current technical and conceptual means.[39] Why would her unconscious wish to change, if indeed she had such a wish, not be expressed biologically? Where else but in her body would this change be taking place? The coma had been induced by a sudden hypoglycemia; it had been an acute organic crisis, a neurobiological and biochemical event of some magnitude, causally connected to her diabetes. It was not clear what mechanisms were involved in the aftermath of this coma, where the pathology was, and where was the even faint promise of repair. Certainly, Vanessa had left behind a part of herself, seemingly in order to recover her younger, slimmer, healthier body, through processes that escaped the bounds of official neurology.

Even if there were an authentic neurological pathology, what was at play here was the regulation through memory of emotions and conflicts, as the psychiatrist put it: her needs were primarily psychological, and so all the doctors could do was recommend her for psychological counselling. She needed to re-define herself in time, through time, from within her body.

The convoluted tale of a life is not the same as the tale of a neuropsychiatric pathology. These twists and turns are a part of the anamnesis – the recorded memory – with which doctors work, and which is all they have before examining the patient. Only after the clinical examination of the fully embodied person does the initial anamnesis become fleshed out, quite literally, along with images of that person's brain, neuropsychological test results, and in some cases biological tests. The difficulty is in making all this information fit together – and if one fails, to try to understand what that failure means and where the free rider is, if there is one. Sometimes, one can only infer the story, especially when the given chronology isn't clear enough for a straightforward diagnostic process. This was the case with Vanessa: there was no *medical* clarity here. The clinical exam was inconclusive. The scans said little. The doctors were aware that the truth did not reside within any of the data they had enlisted. The truth here resided somewhere within Vanessa's embodied mind, body–mind. It might reside in a biological issue that partook of a different body system than the brain, one whose *impact* was neurological – as can happen with diagnoses of functional disease.[40] It may also have partaken of a set of neurological events that were not visible via brain imaging, because no one knew where to look.

It occurred to me that the clinical act is one in which a person probes another, selflessly, discretely in search of a way in – and so that medical knowledge partakes of an act of love of sorts. An anamnesis tells a story that is in part produced by the patient, who usually believes his or her medical narrative is coherent, and whose life gives clues to its meanings. It provides a strangely intimate view of a perfect stranger, like a one-way mirror in an interrogation room. It embraces multiple perspectives – medical episodes, family histories, social circumstances, previous examinations, test results, diagnoses, divergent chronological accounts. It is a proper history – a written memory that is open to reinterpretation, for the doctors must read between its lines, taking nothing for granted, questioning like detectives. It is also a quest for names, for the labels that identify syndromes and diseases. The doctor's role is to find the real medical story, the underlying, invisible coherence that may sometimes be obfuscated by the patient's tale, or sometimes by the specialized nature of medicine itself.

I felt at times that I had heard facts I had no business to know. But these facts never revealed the whole story about the people who came into the room to talk about their ailments and answer questions posed by a benevolent doctor, in front of silently sitting strangers. The person is usually far less fragile, and always far more substantial, in the flesh than on paper. The circuitry of the self, and the byways of a lived life, are hard to untangle even for the finest observers of the brain's byways. Vanessa would probably find resolution, re-connect her twenty-eight-year-old and thirty-eight-year-old selves, and eventually untangle her inner circuitry even without understanding what had happened, rejoining the ranks of all the ordinary people who are unaware of how they remember, and how they forget.

When forgetting is as radical as it is in the case of dementia, most of the anamnesis precedes the onset of the disease. The disease itself is lost in a black hole. My mother is mostly unaware of having remembered, and of forgetting. Unlike Vanessa, she is not on the ball. Anything but. And I sometimes wonder: what is there on the other side of a person whose bearings no longer correspond to those that most of us, most of the time, take for granted? Where has my mother gone? She has no identity amnesia either. She is still herself, a self I still recognize as her – her cool hands, her soft cheeks, her smell and her voice. But she no longer follows the cognitive and linguistic paths of the conversations and temporal signposts we have always unthinkingly shared. The language I can share with her is increasingly limited. To her confusion I can only respond with silence, or dissimulating acquiescence, to spare her the truth of her condition which she cannot understand in any case. I lose my own bearings as a daughter by accepting the loss of hers as a person who otherwise still feels herself, fully, to be my mother. She thinks she is normal. Or rather, her normality is this state that is so strange for everyone around her.

The unawareness of one's own state of illness is called anosognosia (the privative Greek *a* followed by *nosos*, disease, and *gnosos*, knowledge). It is the absence of knowledge about absence, disturbance or incapacity. Vanessa was not anosognosic: on the contrary, she fully grasped her story. She was young and able still. Anosognosia is typical of some people afflicted with dementia like my mother, especially Alzheimer's: according to one theory, it is an aspect of a 'loss of an updated representation of the self'.[41] When embarking on this project, I had initially thought the book should be about anosognosia generally, which, used loosely and not within its clinical context, I believed could be considered descriptive of the human condition – since all of us are somewhat unaware of what ails us most centrally, and much of the time live within our own, neurotic blind spot. Stretching this idea, one could say that dementia is also part of the human condition. One must, simply, accept its occurrence. Sometimes, my mother steps out of the fully anosognosic state for a few seconds into a brief instant of partial lucidity: at those moments she suspects, vaguely, that something is amiss, and becomes furious with a world that is there to fool her and to treat her as a madwoman. Yes she can travel, she can find work, she can set the table, she should learn how to drive. No, Mummy, you can't. Even if it remains anchored within one's self-perception, and however much Vanessa too may have wished otherwise, our youth diminishes – and then it is gone.

4

Haunted

The graves in Jerusalem are gates
of deep tunnels on the day of their opening –
after which they stop digging.

The tombstones are beautiful
cornerstones of buildings
that will never be built.

Yehuda Amichai (trans. with Ted Hughes),
from 'Patriotic Songs' (1978), 18, in *Selected Poems*

As we grow older, the nature of our family heritage comes to the fore, and it may become the stuff of historical memory. It is our responsibility to curate it. But that memory is also embedded in individual memory. And it is too late now for me to ask my mother about much of her early youth, some of which she managed to write about in her memoirs – a messy manuscript stored multiple times on her computer. Her past is distant from that of a Paris-raised, secular person like myself, that much is clear, though there is also a story of uprootedness which continues with me, and which she shared with my father. He was born to a German-speaking, secular Jewish family in Bukovina – an erstwhile, eastern province of the old Austro-Hungarian Empire, divided since the empire's fall in 1919 between Romania and Ukraine. In 1941, he and his family were deported to a Nazi camp, along with all the Jews of the area. His drawings depicting the horrors he saw were what saved him when the (Jewish) capo of the camp saw them: via a deal brokered by the Red Cross exchanging Jewish children for trucks for the Wehrmacht, these drawings enabled his passage in 1944 to British Mandate Palestine, where he finished his adolescence on a kibbutz, studied at Bezalel art school, fought in 1948 (and almost died), then came to Paris, a painter's dream destination.

My mother was actually born in British Mandate Palestine, in the Old City of Jerusalem, into a very religious family that had emigrated to the so-called Holy Land from somewhere in the so-called Pale of Settlement in the Russian Empire in the late eighteenth century. The history was vague, the ancestry mostly unknown. My mother claimed that a great rabbi called the Rabbi of Berdichev was amongst her ancestors. (She still remembers him when I ask her. But then: 'The people who work, they know who it is. The fellow who takes care of all those messages.') They had first gone to Tzvat, the city of mystics. By the time of my mother's birth, in 1932, they had been Jerusalemites for at least five generations. The family was poor. My grandfather, a man with a long beard I have seen in one photograph, and in a drawing by my father which still hangs in my mother's long-unused study, made the crossing to the US before his family. He would return regularly, insemi-nate my grandmother, then go back to New York, where he had settled. It was 1939 and my mother was nearly seven years old when she and the rest of the family joined him. She had two older brothers and one younger one. (They have all since died.) She used to speak Hebrew and Yiddish at home – she occasionally claimed there was also some Arabic, but we aren't sure – then English, which became her language, and hence that of her daughters. They summered in the Catskills, amongst a tight-knit religious community, and not so long ago she was still reminiscing about the idyllic times she had there, with people now long gone. Recently, she said she wanted to call a girl called Rosa she played with there, did I not know her?

She managed to free herself from her religious background, and with the support of her brothers persuade her parents she should study in an ordinary school in New York. She entered City College as an undergraduate in its heyday. A slim-waisted, petite, and beautiful young woman, she danced, had boyfriends, taught rough kids in Harlem. She was part of the Labor Zionist movement. She did an MA at Sarah Lawrence College, and became a poet, although she never dared call herself one, as if it was somehow hubristic – as if a poet was an unreachable divinity. She met my father in Paris, on a trip through Europe, and stayed on. Too typically of her generation, she worked in his shadow. We spoke English in the family – French was the language I spoke, and still speak, with my sister. There was some Hebrew too. I know about the feeling of displacement. It is not dramatic, it can even confer a marvellous freedom, but it is impossible ever to shake off.

Many of the patients I saw were, somehow, displaced, culturally as well as psychologically. Some came from backgrounds that seemed as distant from my own as that of my mother. So it was with Toussaint. 'I was bewitched,' he claimed when he entered the room. 'I have friends back home who are jealous of me.' He had the pleasant, open face of someone who would never harm anyone, and seemed poised when he entered the room. (I won't recount the anamnesis here, as Toussaint's words and the examination tell the story.) He was a Haitian who had lived in France for many years, a married father of four in his late fifties, trained as a plumber and presently unemployed. He had last worked as a school caretaker, and had changed employers repeatedly, as he kept on being fired for being a 'danger to himself and his environment', as how it had been reported. The last time he was fired, he said, was after he had been accused of raking leaves near the gym. When Toussaint told us this story, he displayed a measure of outrage. 'As if raking leaves posed a danger to anyone!' He could not see himself as dangerous. He was a good man, he told us. Religious, too – he knew the evil of the world, and awaited redemption, true to his faith as a Jehovah's Witness. And he knew the boss wanted to replace him with his nephew. It was blatantly unfair. Yet revenge was not the way. God would see to it that justice was done. He, Toussaint, had never wished to harm anyone. But he was upset. And anxious.

Prompted by the doctor, he told us why he was seeking professional help. Over the past three years or so, he said, his nights had become bad. He suffered from sleep apnea, so much so that he had a machine to counter the countless interruptions in breathing he experienced in his sleep. But he still woke all the time. And he dreamed a lot, so even when he did sleep through without waking, he was never rested enough: 'I have the impression of sleeping without sleeping,' was how he put it. He was so sleep deprived that, he confessed, 'I wonder how I can hold on. Sometimes I think I won't survive.' He would take naps during the day, but those weren't effective. He managed diurnal life by remaining active – reading, listening to the radio. But he had developed trouble concentrating. And making decisions. He had also been caught speeding a few times, though he had not realized he was over the limit on those occasions. His wife found him forgetful and moody. He often felt sad, though twenty-five years had passed since he'd been diagnosed with proper depression. In any case, as far as he was concerned, his main problem was that he was haunted. He heard things.

There were whisperings. And presences. They had started a dozen years back. And they had grown worse over the past few years, after he had built himself a small house. He was pretty sure he knew what they were – and who: the higher status he had reached upon becoming a house owner, however small and modest the house, had triggered envy in some of his friends in Haiti, and now they were persecuting him. So far away, and so close. There they were, in his head, invading him when he was alone and just trying to mind his own business. They wouldn't leave him be. Day and night. And each day, as he was waking up, in that halfway place between sleep and wakefulness, the land of nightmares awaited him. He started hearing sounds such as menacing cracks, voices, unintelligible words – and a force assaulted him. He would try to get up to defend himself but couldn't. He felt the force attempt to strangle him. He would try to cry out – and his wife would shake him awake, if she was there. The assault would only stop once he was fully awake, sometimes after what seemed like a long time. And this happened every day. Even on holiday. The voices were there in the background, constantly – his daytime nightmares. And all the more so since he'd moved into his little house.

Toussaint told his story calmly and lucidly, even rationally. Despite the anxiety with which he lived, he had found a way to accommodate that unpleasant, constant company, and to accept it. It was par for the course, he said: he was not the first and certainly not the last to experience *maraboutage*, as his Haitian countrymen called it. The African, and thence Haitian *marabout* is a seer, sometimes healer, sometimes witch, and Toussaint felt he was the victim of this traditional sorcery, persecuted by the spirits. As he told the psychiatrist in the room, the fact that his wife liked 'old furniture' made it all the likelier, in his mind, that spirits could haunt their house. But he loved life, he told us, raising his voice a little. And his faith stood strong against that profane force. He prayed in order to make the voices go away, and it usually worked. His family and friends sustained him too. He told us that he believed the sorcery had begun much earlier, when he was still a boy in Haiti and had moved houses with his parents: he remembered the tell-tale lights that once passed through the new house, bewitching it. According to the lore, if someone inside was 'touched' by these lights, that person was effectively bewitched as well – *marabouté* is the word for this. His brother was touched by the lights, and he had died very young, at the age of eighteen. There was a coherence here, thought Toussaint. He admitted he had no 'rational certainty' about this, and he himself would never resort to witchcraft in any case, because it clashed with his faith. But yes, he knew that he was bewitched.

On the other hand, he told us with an amused smile, his wife thought he was 'ill in the head'. On her insistence, he had previously consulted a psychiatrist who told him he was afflicted with a 'persecution complex' and suggested hypnosis as a possible healing method, though, Toussaint said, hypnosis would also be at odds with his faith, so he didn't go down that route. There was a brief silence. Then the psychiatrist in the room proposed: 'We have the impression that even if you have enemies, you're suffering more than necessary, so we'll try to help you.' The doctor suggested that medicine could help Toussaint, because it could be that he was imagining some things, out of anxiety. Toussaint agreed that if indeed this was an illness, and if indeed he was imagining things – well then, maybe medicine would help. There was a haunting, certainly, but he needed all the support he could get.

Even though doctors are trained to see and listen without judgement, it took a particularly empathic understanding on their part, I soon felt, to listen to Toussaint's story on its own terms – and one may say that medicine at its best is also the practice of cultural empathy. It was clearly important for the medical team to consider his beliefs in order to understand how he felt. And in turn, he seemed quite content to deliver himself over to their medical scrutiny and care. As the examination proceeded, it emerged that he had other symptoms, of which he only complained in passing, unaware that, to a clinical eye, they carried significance and were signs pointing to a pathology. His balance was a little off, for instance: he didn't walk as steadily as he used to. Then there was the neuropsychological evaluation: an extensive series of tests that help identify and rate on a precise scale a person's cognitive and perceptual capacities, the results of which are always read out with the anamnesis, before patients come into the room. It had emerged from these tests that Toussaint displayed a deficit in attention span, and that he had a 'dysexecutive and attentional syndrome': he did not reason clearly and had trouble remaining focused on one task without getting distracted. The tests also revealed that his social cognition was subpar, meaning that he did not interpret social clues as one ordinarily does, and that his recognition of emotions in others was slightly off – he failed to recognize a person's expression of fear in a picture, for instance. Tested in the room, under our eyes, Toussaint had trouble naming pictures of animals and recognizing objects including a screwdriver, which was odd for a plumber. In other words, he was not interpreting the world quite as clearly as it seemed from his self-presentation. When tested on recognition of animals, he named a lion a wolf, a ladybird a toad, a lobster an insect, a squirrel a rabbit, and an owl a parrot. 'In my country I did pretty lousy studies and wasn't used to images,' he justified himself, slightly embarrassed.

Toussaint also was experiencing a change in his ability to enjoy things in life, he told us: he had always loved music, for instance, but now he had stopped listening. He wanted to feel joy and enjoy music again. He would do what it took. The psychiatrist said his seemed a case of 'anhedonia' – the inability to experience pleasure, which was itself most often a symptom of depression. The term anhedonia was coined by Théodule Ribot, the insightful psychologist we met earlier.[1] Its Greek etymology gives us 'absence of joy', *hedonè*. (The first time I heard the term was when, a long time ago, my mother discovered it, paradoxically delighted at such a beautiful sounding name for something as sad as the loss of the ability to feel pleasure.) The neurologist suggested to Toussaint that this anhedonia could have been due to lack of sleep, or, conversely, that he lacked sleep because of it. Toussaint was taking anti-depressants, in fact, and it was possible, suggested the doctor, that these were also playing a part in inducing his nightmares.

In any case, it was clear that, somehow, his dreaming life had seeped into his waking life and vice versa, just as, conversely, his dreams had become terribly real.[2] Toussaint's interpretation of this frightening experience fits neatly into a story allowed and favoured by Haitian culture: he was being persecuted by outside, occult forces whose intent was malicious. But the scientific fact of the matter was that those forces came from within, and the voices he heard during the day to be those of enemies from back home were, in clinical terms, auditory verbal hallucinations – AVH for short.

A hallucination is a fairly common phenomenon. Oliver Sacks devoted a book to it, *Hallucinations*.[3] Esquirol, the psychiatrist we met earlier, who was initially mentored by Pinel at La Salpêtrière, famously defined it as a 'perception without an object' in his treatise on mental illnesses, published in 1838.[4] Today we generally understand a hallucination as the outcome of a surge of activity in the cerebral area that is usually involved in the perceptual processes related to those sounds, visions or sensations, that emerge in the absence of a real object.[5] A hallucination can occur for each sense, or modality: during a hallucination, you somehow sense – see, hear, taste or feel – something that others around you do not perceive. Esquirol calls the hallucinator a 'visionary' in this respect.[6] Hallucinations are not always the sign of a mental illness.[7] They can occur in the form of the aura preceding a migraine, or be induced through the taking of drugs; they can occur as the re-enaction of trauma in PTSD, as a manifestation of grief, from

sleep-deprivation, or in situations of prolonged sensory deprivation – for instance, images can appear if one stares for a
long time at a blank wall, or becomes blind.[8] And one can
'hear voices' while being perfectly sane.[9] Sacks even wonders
'why most of us do not hear voices'. He conjectures that what
enables us not to attribute external agency to inner voices may
be a construct, what he calls a 'physiological barrier or inhibition'.[10] (More on this later.) One can hallucinate whole pieces
of music. A voice can emerge from within, but as if from
without, in situations of stress or extreme danger. In all such
cases, one remains aware of the hallucinatory nature of the
experience: they are known as 'critiqued' hallucinations, and
they can come in the form of 'thought insertions'.[11]

But Toussaint did not have such an awareness: he did not
conceive of his voices as hallucinations. Such unawareness –
such anosognosia – is usually the sign of a mental pathology
of some sort. Once Toussaint left the room, and discussion of
his case began, the doctors surmised that his hallucinations
were an aspect of what they agreed was some sort of 'delirium',
which they believed was connected to his depression, his sleep
disturbances and his bad dreams. The etymology of the Latin
denotes deviation (*de*) from a ridge between furrows (*lira*), from
a straight line. In a state of delirium, one is literally de-ranged:
subjective experience of sense-perceptions and sensations is not
in line with actual inputs. Many conditions can produce delirium
and any associated hallucinations; these may be short-lived or
chronic, non-pathological or, indeed, indicative of a serious
condition. What was Toussaint's condition, then?

The interpretation of any symptom is called a medical 'semiology', since the symptoms to be interpreted are *signs* of a
condition, and these signs need to be read, like a text. The
semiology is spelt out in precise names for symptoms that correspond to particular cerebral deficits – verbally smoothed-out
impediments that belie strange or harsh realities. The names

were created for the most part from the nineteenth century on, out of ancient Greek, monosyllabic prefixes and suffixes that name the alteration or loss of faculties we take for granted: *arthron*, articulation; *tonos*, tension; *praxis*, action; *kinesis*, motion; *gnosos*, knowledge; *mnesis*, memory; *lexis*, speech; *osmê*, smell; *boulè*, will; *phasis*, phase; *thumós*, soul. There is the *dys* of abnormality or impairment – its 'y' echoing its Sanskrit origin meaning bad, or difficult. There is the *a* privative in Sanskrit and in Greek. The prefixes yield a myriad of conditions that are sometimes difficult to imagine, let alone comprehend, from an ordinary, non-clinical perspective – and some of which are reported in these pages: dysarthria, slurred speech; dystonia, muscular spasms that impede voluntary motion; dyspraxia, bad coordination; apraxia, difficulty in accomplishing movements; akynesia, loss of ability to initiate voluntary movement; agnosia, loss of ability to recognize things presented to us by our senses; amnesia, loss of memory; alexia, loss of ability to recognize written words; anosmia, loss of sense of smell; abulia, loss of motivation; aphasia, an impairment in linguistic expression or comprehension; alexithymia, difficulty in feeling and recognizing emotions. These can be irreversible losses, though some abilities and states can be recovered too, the prefixes kicked away.

The semiology depends on what information is available, and on the underlying cultural and scientific assumptions and beliefs about the nature of the illness: medical vocabulary changes as data and interpretive theories change. The semiology in Toussaint's case included hallucinations, delirium, and depression. States like his have been described throughout the history of modern psychiatry. The notion of delirium comes up centrally in the respective nosologies – classifications of disease – of Pinel and Esquirol. Pinel believed that delirium was an aspect of what he called *vésanie* – a term that he borrowed from the English 'vesania', translatable at first as insanity and, from 1850 onwards, as psychosis.[12] At first, he had divided these *vésanies* into four broad categories: hysteria and hypochondria, encountered earlier, and mania and melancholia, two conditions which had been paired for centuries.[13] In a later classification, one of the four orders of *vésanies* was that of hallucinations – and mania and melancholia were also associated with delirium.[14] Esquirol would soon after divide melancholia into what he called 'monomania' and 'lypemania';[15] today it corresponds to a combination of psychotic delirium and depression.[16]

Was Toussaint's case a vesania, then? Was he psychotic? If so, how, and why? The semiology only named a state and pointed at possible causes; it did not describe it. So what was this internal state of his that meant he felt so terribly persecuted, menaced, sleep-deprived, and joyless? The interpretation of his case turned out to be rather more complex than had first appeared. And this complexity, I realized as I thought about it, was due in part to the long history of the very phenomenon of hallucination. The term itself, whose etymology points to the Latin *alucinari* – which means to wander in the mind, to ramble, to dream – was coined by the famous physician Sir Thomas Browne, in 1646, two centuries before Esquirol turned it into a psychiatric pathology.[17] Before then, voices and visions of this kind were endowed with a religious significance, and were interpreted as messages from gods or devils, or ancestral spirits. They were associated with dreams, with the powers of prophecy, creativity, and inspiration. The modern association of hallucination with delirium, madness and, today in particular, schizophrenia, has overwhelmed these earlier cultural connotations.[18] Yet Toussaint's experience harked back to them, as well as manifesting as a disorder within his organism.

To begin with the biological disorder. It was significant that Toussaint had trouble sleeping, and that his dreaming life was so very rich, because of the association of dreams with visions that are also the hallmark of hallucinations. The neurologist suggested that, as Toussaint woke continuously throughout most nights, often in the midst of dream-rich REM (rapid eye movement) sleep, he had a higher chance of remembering his dreams, giving him the feeling that his waking life was invaded by nightmares.[19] Our diurnal and nocturnal cognitive lives are complementary, and dreams arguably fulfill the function of pruning memory, of reorganizing cognitive inputs and structures, and elaborating emotional states and responses. And when awake, we normally differentiate remembered dreams from remembered, actual, events. But in Toussaint's case, the distinction between night and day was blurred, and his dreams were continuously becoming part of his episodic, autobiographical memory: he remembered them as if they were memories of real events.

Much about the mechanisms of sleep and dreaming remains unknown to researchers. One can safely say that dreams are, at least in part, elaborations of sensory experiences and salient thoughts, interactions and emotions that have occurred during the day, a cocktail of thoughts, visual impressions and sounds that are chaotically re-activated during sleep - in the words of philosopher Suzanne Langer, the brain's translation of 'experiences into symbols, in fulfilment of a basic need to do so'.[20] And one could further hypothesize that when we recall those dreams after waking up we are weaving bits of oneiric activity together into a legible, memorable narrative. By remembering and retelling a dream narrative, we *create* the very meaning we may be looking for in what, during sleep, were chaotic, jumbled sequences. Those dreams in which there is no awareness that one is dreaming, no suspension of disbelief so to speak – for there are also 'lucid dreams' in which the dreamer knows it is all a dream – are the sleeping equivalents of hallucinations in wakefulness.[21] So in some way, Toussaint was injecting into his oneiric visions a narrative that made sense to him, and that translated also, in his waking life, as hallucinations. Esquirol had described how a hallucinator 'dreams awake': the dreamer processes the previous day's ideas during sleep, while a person in a state of delirium 'finishes the dream after waking up. Dreams, like hallucinations, always reproduce old ideas.'[22]

In both dream and hallucination, I am at once here and somewhere else. My body constructs an experience that is anchored in sensorimotor mechanisms, events and impressions encoded in memory, while also being dissociated from sensorimotor inputs. It is a paradoxical state, lived in two parallel dimensions. Toussaint's experience, such as we could make it out from his description, combined elements from processes involved in both sleep and hallucination. It consisted of a rich layering of emotions, memories, oneiric free association – the type of strange narratives and layerings present in dreams – and dysfunctions that distorted his sensory experiences and his relation to external reality. Throughout, the voices were a constant, as was the story he understood them to be a part of. In all phenomena of acoustic hallucinations, one perceives self-generated thoughts as voices, as if one were no longer the agent of one's own thoughts. The sense of agency, in effect, is disturbed, as it was disturbed in Toussaint's case: sounds, visions, impressions, sensations fabricated out of memory processes are no longer experienced as originating from or pertaining to the self.[23] In schizophrenia it is typical to attribute an external, sometimes malevolent agency to external objects (such as televisions) and to sounds that are in fact generated from within.[24] Hearing voices, however, is just one aspect of a diagnosis of schizophrenia. Toussaint's AVH were specifically tied into his sleep disturbances, meshing with oneiric life, and he did not display any other symptoms of schizophrenia.

One way in which hallucinatory experiences differ from imagination is in their realism: the mind creates its own reality. This is why there often remains a conviction even in the most rational of patients that there is *something real* about their hallucination.

Toussaint was one of those: he was convinced that he had been bewitched. During the discussion of his case, the neurologist who had examined him mentioned a patient he had seen years before, who was convinced he had implants in his retina, regardless of the fact that no implants could be seen on imaging. He also recalled another patient who was sure that a witch doctor from back home had put an object in his head, and wondered whether it would be visible on a brain scan. 'If you tell a schizophrenic patient they're hearing voices, that confirms their delirium!' quipped the psychiatrist. A persecution complex is so potent precisely because anything and everything is interpreted by the patient as evidence of persecution, in a form of extreme confirmation bias – so that even its refutation by a seemingly benevolent doctor is perceived as persecution, serving to confirm its reality. Toussaint felt persecuted. But even if we do not hear menacing voices, we all experience variations in how we experience reality, because perception itself is such a complex phenomenon. And as Oliver Sacks had noted in *Hallucinations*,[25] AVH experiences are fairly common in part because of the ways in which we construct our ordinary experience of the world in the first place.[26]

For we do *construct* our experience – we do not passively receive and process perceptual information. We are not information processing machines. We actively generate our relation to the environment we are embedded in. To understand this, it helps to take a few steps away from that clinical room and its patients, away from the case of Toussaint, and into the broader realm of our biological history. And we can look at how 'the body is a foundation of the conscious mind,' as neurologist Antonio Damasio put it: our brains serve our bodies, rather than the other way round.[27] Consider then, with Damasio, that we descend from early life forms consisting of single-cell organisms and bacteria, devoid of a nervous system though engaged in sensing, and responding to, the environment, and in basic motor action. These single cells evolved into multicellular systems of increasing complexity, eventually endowed with nervous systems that coordinated multiple organ systems and their intercommunication. We can then conceive of our sophisticated brain as precisely the evolved mechanism that enables us to engage in action and perception, and to ensure the regulation of 'homeostasis' – the mechanism thanks to which we are able to survive within the always changing environment. Homeostasis is what ensures that an organism's physiology – such as heart rate, temperature, metabolism, and so on – remains within viable bounds. Our inherently homeostatic selves are on a continuum with the homeostatically governed single cells and bacteria from which all complex organisms evolved.[28] And to homeostasis corresponds 'allostasis', which is the anticipatory adjustment that the organism engages in to achieve homeostatic stability. We would die if we were unable to *anticipate* how environmental temperature influences body temperature, and so adjust our actions accordingly – drink when thirsty, or swim in the cool sea when the sun is hot, say.[29]

It is from computational neuroscience that there has emerged a way to explain *how* this anticipation happens, how an organism endowed with agency survives through environmental changes, maintaining itself within its viable homeostatic range and responding to external cues in a way appropriate to its survival: the theory of 'predictive processing'. First posited by UCL neuroscientist Karl Friston about a decade ago, and developed also by philosopher Andy Clark, who integrated Friston's predictive processing into his own theories about embodied cognition, this theory is of such explanatory power that it has become hugely influential. As Friston puts it, 'We are thrown into the world as a process already in motion; and processes can only reason towards what is "out there" based on sparse (if carefully selected) samples of the world.'[30] And so, the brain is an inherently predictive organ that responds to constant internal or environmental changes by *predicting* sensory information on the basis of previous instances, much as a statistical machine would do.[31] In Friston's terms, for an organism to maintain itself within certain physiological bounds – within a viable homeostatic range – it must avoid or at least minimize 'surprises'.[32] And the brain does so by 'generating predictions to explain sensory states'.[33] When it encounters stimuli, whether these are external or internal to the organism, it generates its own explanations for them, testing the hypotheses it has built – from its birth onward – against incoming sensations.[34] (Think of how you expect a glass of water to have a certain weight when you grab it – and the surprise you feel if the weight is less than expected, leading your hand to fly up.) The brain develops in such a way that it becomes able to *infer* the causes of a sensation or perception, in a Bayesian, inferential mechanism that has come to be called 'predictive coding'. Any discrepancy between its 'top-down' prediction, or 'prior expectations', and the 'bottom-up' signal or new sensory evidence, is a 'prediction error'. A resulting state of health is one in which this error has been corrected. A state of illness, or one of emotional distress, or psychic or cognitive dysfunction, is one in which we are unable to correct the erroneous expectation.

Such an understanding of perceptual and cognitive processes does a lot to explain what may be happening in a hallucination, that is, how one may misattribute the causes of a perception.[35] And it also can help account for psychosis: 'Mismatches between prior beliefs and incoming signals constitute prediction errors that drive new learning. Psychosis has been suggested to result from a decreased precision in the encoding of prior beliefs relative to the sensory data, thereby garnering maladaptive inferences,' according to one recent study.[36] A hallucination, whether it is caused by psychosis or not, is here on a continuum with a simple sensory illusion: both arise out of faulty signalling in relation to our own predictions, so that we mistake our expectations for reality. Toussaint's terrible haunting and delirium could be interpreted as an instance of this. An AVH is a delusion – as Esquirol named it – a misattribution of agency, an aberrant perception that translates as disturbed cognition.[37] In predictive processing terms, it is a massive, uncorrected prediction error, a case of those prior expectations having much more weight than incoming sensory information.[38] This theory was not discussed within the clinical setting. But even if it had been, how would it have helped Toussaint get better? And how would it account for his narcolepsy, and his disturbed REM sleep, as well as his persistent anhedonia? There was also his difficulty in recognizing objects and animals. The neurologist brought up during the discussion of his case the possibility that this latter symptom could be due to herpetic encephalitis – a lesion in the temporal lobe caused by an infection of the brain by the virus of the herpes family – though the hypothesis would require testing and further imaging.[39]

Another element may come into play here. As the doctor pointed out, Toussaint's hallucinations were narcoleptic: they manifested as 'REM sleep intrusions', a dream-like state in the middle of apparent wakefulness, a disturbance in REM sleep known as RBD, for REM Behaviour Disorder.[40] And such narcoleptic hallucinations, where the diurnal and nocturnal overlap and fuse in the strange way Toussaint experienced, were often indicative of Parkinson's disease. Parkinson's is notably characterized by a decline in the availability of the neurotransmitter dopamine, which plays a central role in initiating movement (hence the tremor typical of the disease in humans). Dopamine is found in many living organisms, and is essential in ensuring that the agent's response to internal or environmental cues is appropriate – it is even active in plants' regulation of circadian rhythms.[41] Recent studies show that dopamine – released within a part of the brain associated with reward and decision-making called the striatum – also plays a

role in the integration of sensory evidence with sensory predictions, and that an *excess* of it is associated with hallucinations.[42]
It would be difficult to ascertain how exactly the dopaminergic
system was playing out in Toussaint's syndrome, but something
there was awry – particularly with regard to his disordered
circadian rhythm.[43] The doctors all agreed that RBD was
present in his case, however, and that the sleep deprivation
would account for his anhedonia as well. The psychiatrist also
went over the medications Toussaint was already taking – these
included an anti-psychotic, which, he told us, might be
enhancing the anxiety and even causing the nightmares.
Toussaint needed a better anti-depressant, and an alternative
anti-psychotic for his delirium. The neurologist completed
these recommendations: a sleep report to establish RBD, an
investigation of his visual recognition issues, a lumbar puncture
(abbreviated to LP) to search for biomarkers in the cerebrospinal fluid, and a so-called DaTscan to look for Parkinson's.[44]

By the end of the discussion of Toussaint's case, diagnosis was
suspended. And as I only saw each patient once, without ever
recording their names, I was not able to follow up what
emerged from the tests. One could only hope medication
would help him, and that his voices would leave him in peace.
But a 'whodunnit' of disease could not sum up Toussaint's
experience, which was part of that long cultural history of
hallucination I was thinking about as I observed his examination. And Toussaint's cultural background gave the complex
biological processes that produced his symptoms a specific
content and tenor.

This background was one in which the reality of a spirit
world was writ large. The doctors who examined him had been
attentive to his way of telling his story for that reason, careful
to take seriously his convictions.[45] Theirs was an anthropological stance of sorts, in which, for the time of the examination

of their patient, they stepped outside their secular, scientific frame of reference, and accepted the centrality to the hallucinator's experience of the spirit world which was integral to his sense of cultural belonging. For that hour, they listened as would a sorcerer, a shaman, or a priest. From ancient Greece to medieval Europe, clerics were often doctors. In ancient Greece, it was believed that Aesculapius, the god of medicine, healed patients who spent the night at his temples by visiting them in their dreams, in the form of a serpent.[46] In all cultures, illness is a state that marks the boundary between life and death, and so religious energy is intensely focused on that liminal state. By extension, the doctor as shaman, seer, sorcerer or priest is the recipient of visions from a dream-like realm beyond the present, and beyond the here and now of natural laws and chronological time, endowed with a force that can act upon and subvert nature.

It isn't clear what exactly Toussaint was expecting of the doctors whose rule and role he so benevolently accepted. But what occurred to me that day was that I was witnessing in his examination an ancient ritual, not just a medical consultation with a psychotic patient. He was someone for whom, as for millions before him, throughout human history and in all cultures, hallucination and dream belong to the other side of daily life and give meaning. He was able to reconcile acceptance of his bewitchment as a reality with his official faith, via the – hallucinatory – power of the unseen. It is worth recalling that ancient interpretations of dreams have always seen them as potential prophesies. In the Sumerian, 4,000-year-old *Epic of Gilgamesh*, the eponymous hero dreams of the arrival of his future friend Enkidu. In the Old Testament, the prophetic potency of Joseph's dreams of power causes his brothers to sell him to the Egyptians – while his capacity to interpret accurately the dreams of others as prophesies leads Pharaoh to hand him the governance of Egypt. In one of the most famous treaties of dream interpretation, the second-century *Oneirocritica* of the Ephesan Artemidorus, dreams are meaningful insofar as they foretell the future, while ever since the publication of Freud's *Interpretation of Dreams*, in 1900, they have tended to be seen as signifying one's emotionally laden relation to the past or present.[47]

Dreams are like doors to the non-present, the not-here, not-now, an escape from linear time – seemingly an escape from the body. They are a liminal process, like illness itself. Unlike the stone out of which we have carved our immortal gods, mortal, living creatures vitally need sleep. We humans have a dream world that is integral to our cognitive make-up, in that it allows us to work through our thoughts, emotions and experiences. It is all the more fascinating that fatigue, and not just psychosis, can lead to cognitive illusions. To interpret such illusions as visions from an extra-corporeal realm contradicts biological accounts, and requires a belief in a separation between soul and body. Such a separation was first advanced in the West by Plato – who lived when the Greek gods were still potent, their stone statues still venerated, and the Sybils, those flesh-and-blood prophetesses of the ancient world, still spoke in their name. And this separation of soul and body sustains religious faith. The great fourteenth-century Arab historian and philosopher Ibn Khaldun devoted pages of his *Muqaddimah* to the nature of dreams and what gives them prophetic power: 'The soul,' he writes, 'becomes spiritual through freeing itself from bodily matters and corporeal perceptions. This happens to the soul in the form of glimpses through the agency of sleep,' whereby it 'gains the knowledge of future events that it desires'. Dreams give us access to the 'high spiritual world and the essences it contains, from visions and things we had not been aware of while awake but which we find in our sleep and which are brought to our attention in it and which, if dreams are true, conform with actuality.'

There can be 'confused dreams' as well, which are 'pictures of the imagination stored inside by perception and to which the ability to think is applied'. And so, if chosen, and virtuous, the sleeper can be the recipient of divine messages, rather than just a person whose imagination is active in sleep.[48]

Oneiric visions have a hallucinatory reality in these descriptions, transmitting messages from a supernatural realm, beyond that of ordinary, linear, spatio-temporally-bound experience. Midway between wakefulness and the unconscious dream state, they are passageways that explain and determine diurnal reality and their bearers become messengers. But the messages Toussaint heard were all menace, envy, negativity – and meant for him only, it seemed. He had no one to transmit them to. They were the sign *of* illness rather than messages *about* an illness that he could share with a sorcerer for relief. One might even surmise that part of his difficulty was his separation from a society where his visitations would make sense.[49] For oneiric and hallucinatory experiences are central to the social and religious life of many cultures. The voices heard collectively in such states can infuse individual dreams, collective tales or waking life, and are deliberately provoked within states of trance induced by repetitive, bodily and sung rhythms and incantations, sometimes assisted by psychotropic substances, from ergot to ayahuasca, the Peruvian plant that has become fashionable amongst Western urbanites.[50] They partake of that liminal realm in which absentees, gods or dead ancestors return and speak to the living. The African, and thence specifically Haitian *marabout* is a seer endowed with the power to welcome these visitors. This is a religion syncretic enough for a Jehovah's Witness such as Toussaint to be able to accept the potency of a *maraboutage* as real, and not in conflict with his stringent, Christian beliefs.

But the job of Western medicine, which began in ancient Greece on terrain shared by priests, remains to subvert the occult. Literally to bring to light what is hidden – occulted – to explain and try to heal the body's travails in naturalistic rather than divine terms, even though its explanations and solutions can be unsatisfying in their mechanistic approach. Its focus is not belief but the event inside the body – which is often at once occulted and brought to light by the patient's testimonial and convictions. A sentence becomes clinically significant only if one has learned how to hear. The good doctor brings knowledge to bear on observations in order to interpret their meaning, to 'arrive at a semiology'.

For there is the person, the patient, and the brain. Each patient whose brain may figure as an image on a computer screen is a person. Each person is someone's child, parent, partner, friend, family member. Only as such do their stories make sense, and only as such do the scans make some sense. The impressive ways in which the doctors try to 'arrive at a semiology' from variegated signs and signals always gives one hope that meaning can be found in all corners, and that it can remain throughout the neural transformations wrought by illness. It is a matter of taking the patient at their word while reading between the lines, remaining aware that the testimonial is at once a real story, a sign, and a potential signal. What was most striking about the case of Toussaint was that it represented a meeting point halfway between evidence and belief, biology and culture, pharmacology and tradition. Modern science makes no room for the transcendent meanings of hallucinatory phenomena. But what became clear that day was that the best treatment in the case of Toussaint was one that reconciled his belief system with the powers of modern medicine and its pharmacopeia – where doctors acknowledged, as do witches, its dangers and its limitations. Only thus, and also with the help of some drugs, would he regain some peace within himself, and within his home.

Regaining peace would also mean reconciling himself with

his past, which was not a straightforward one. As a native Haitian, he was somewhat displaced in France, while also being at home. Like all Haitians, he spoke French because, in the late seventeenth century, French colonists had brutally brought slaves from Africa to work on the sugar plantations that enriched the metropole – and the *maraboutage* of which Toussaint was the victim had been brought to Haiti from Africa as well. Like most Haitians too, indeed like most descendants of colonized people or slaves, he had a heavy, painful inheritance. He was proud of his metropolitan house, which was his permanent abode, even though it may have felt temporary to him, invaded by the insistent presence of a powerful, multi-layered past that called him back. Toussaint's cultural memory was problematic, unresolved. And now that a neuropathology had emerged, it was feeding into his delusions.

While thinking about Toussaint again, and about how central cultural and family memory are to the self, I realize I am trying to salvage my mother's past. For it is fading fast. While Toussaint was coherent in his delusions and waking dreams, my mother manifests incoherence. As memory disintegrates, she no longer connects her present with her past, and her delusions, unlike Toussaint's, are nearly devoid of bygone voices. Toussaint's origins and life are worlds away from hers, or mine. But displacement due to larger historical forces and the global movements of populations are common to both him and each of my parents, who transmitted impermanence to me because of their respective histories, both born as they were in places that no longer exist. My mother's birthplace was colonial territory as well, however long ago her ancestors had arrived in that disputed land. Her subsequent American childhood and youth, for which she harboured, once, some nostalgia, was overshadowed by more than sixty years in Paris. She never fully conquered the French language, and wrote, always, only in English, which she is speaking much more now, even though the women who care for her speak none. She is fully in her present, because she is forgetting where she comes from. But I grew up with the figurative packed suitcase in the corner: we had never planned to stay where we were. Still, stay we did, and I had the luck to grow up in a steady home – still standing, and little changed since my childhood. My father is buried not far away, in the Cimetière du Montparnasse, a Parisian forever. I left France after school (returning to live in Paris only after a good two decades), but my mother has been in that same flat for over fifty years. These days she sometimes calls it a 'hotel'. She is borrowing her space. Or she repeats, sitting in the living room, as I make a move to put on my coat and return to my house after a visit, 'I must go home now.'

A home can be an imaginary construct, as well as an inheritance. Our body needs a home to survive, however impermanent. The mother's body is the embodied self's first home. This, my mother remains for me. She will always be the voice resonating against my cheek as I fell asleep on her chest, a tired child in the cab from Tel Aviv airport to Jerusalem, feeling the Hebrew sounds, basking in the sudden humid heat and smells that struck as soon as we landed in the middle of the night, for our summer holidays. It all felt safe, promising, infinitely loving, and ancestral. She and my father were very much at home there. For me, it was a Mediterranean elsewhere, a sensorial contrast to Parisian greys. Eventually I would mostly leave behind the place that had revealed itself as the impossible, shattered dream it is – though Mediterranean nature remains deep under my skin. But as a child, arrival there always was synonymous with that nocturnal cab trip, my mother speaking the ancient language I only partly own, but which is so familiar and intelligible. The mother's body, and its past: this is where we start from, and it is from here that we can construct all our perceptions, and all our future homes.[51]

5

Appearances

Minds emerge from process and interaction, not substance.
In a sense, we inhabit the spaces between things. We subsist
in emptiness. A beautiful, liberating thought and nothing to
be afraid of. The notion of a tethered soul is crude by
comparison. Shine a light, it's obvious.

Paul Broks, *Into the Silent Land:*
Travels in Neuropsychology (2003)

My mother's embodied self *feels* identical to what it has always
been. When I hug her, I hug *her*. She looks at me in the way
she has always looked at me – and the maternal gaze holds
me in a unique way. The recognition between us remains. She
still knows me. She is still my mother, the woman whose body
I come from, and against which I slept in the cab to Jerusalem.
But neglect of the body's care is one of the terrible effects of
dementia. She continues to dress elegantly, with help. She used
to love perfume, though she lost much of her sense of smell
many years ago, following a fall on her head. (Or was it a
prelude to the dementia? Loss of smell is predictive of it.[1])
She used to put on too much perfume as a result, saying 'it
will go away' if one protested. That is over now. She no longer
remembers to shower. The people who help her, twenty-four
hours a day, are marvels, and saviours. I feel I am too close to
her to be the one to shower her, and care for her as if she

were a child. Both she and I would feel humiliation. I would get too angry, impatient, and baffled: I could not possibly act as anything other than what I have always been – her daughter. (When the child must become the parent, as is often the case, guilt, humiliation and anger can sour a relationship. I am lucky I can entrust her basic care to others in this way.)

For her affect is remarkably intact. She still tries to read people's emotions, including mine. She senses situations to some extent, still can follow stories for a few seconds at least, and remembers, up to a point, where she must be when. She speaks as a woman who has always been a poet through and through – with the poet's wordplay that can dress things up, the 'pathetic fallacies' of the poetic imagination. She is still able to mock herself – a distancing of sorts, though one mostly unknowing of its function. 'How come you look so young?' I asked her recently. 'I do terrible things to my face.' Her state fluctuates still, as I write this. There are moments of cogency. In the meantime, while time unravels her, and while a sentence about her state becomes out of date as fast as fresh milk, all I can do is stand still.

My father often disparaged my mother during their fifty-one years together. We two daughters always had an intensely involved, close relationship with them both, and after his death, we could be short-tempered with her, as if we felt the need to replicate his behaviour. We were irritated with her frequent confusions – irritation is an outgrowth of intimacy, after all. We didn't see it coming: the passage from ordinary confusion to pathology is perversely subtle, and the realization that dementia is on its way is almost always retrospective, so creeping is the progression of this condition. It eludes most family members. At first, quirks of character became exaggerated. What were once amusing or indeed merely irritating slips, confusions and misrememberings, or faults of character, became increasingly bizarre statements, all the more surreal in that they seamlessly wove themselves into a lucid sentence. A semantically fluent conversation, grammatically correct, idiomatically rich, would fill up with entirely inappropriate associations. Conversation continued but made decreasing sense, each day adding another subtle layer of opacity to what, seemingly a long while ago, was a wholly lucid mind. There were overlaps between fragmented impressions, fears and wishes, memories of people, books, films, faces, others' voices, events from one place displaced to another continent and another era – emotionally inflected interpretations of increasingly blurry facts. What, where, when, slipped out of each other's hold, dissolved and re-emerged in new shapes. She would get angry when contradicted, believing that we were set against her. Sometimes she would forcefully find odd meanings in order to maintain within herself a semblance of coherence. Illness declares itself precisely when what was once shared time and shared space stops being unquestionably shared. When it becomes a dividing line.

The line came into view: finally we had to acknowledge the insidiously advancing illness. She was not at fault. She was ill. We had to stop reacting according to the family's old emotional patterns. Of course, she had never been 'at fault', and the previous blame and irritation were not in the least justified either. But now we could no longer express frustration, engage in discussion, hope for improvement, because there was no discussion possible, no grounds for hope, and no possibility of improvement. With the disappearance of those frequent mother–daughter frictions, so intimate and so full of mutual knowledge, there disappeared a whole aspect of our own selves as daughters. It was a new, alienating landscape. The anger with her first shifted to a deep fury at this debilitating condition. Then, acceptance. By now, the new condition has become familiar.

◆

I saw Geraldine at the clinical meeting long before I realized I was the daughter of someone afflicted with impending dementia. Her husband had suffered from advancing Alzheimer's Disease and was living in a facility near her house when he fled one day, in 2002, and never came back. He was registered as a missing person. She was sixty-seven. That was how the anamnesis of Geraldine began, read out by one of the junior doctors on rotation in the unit. But of course it was her own troubles that brought her here. The report went on: she had been depressed since 2000. She had trouble seeing since surgery for melanoma in one eye, and she had an unoperated cataract in the other. She forgot some words, too often for her taste. And over the past few years, she had started experiencing hallucinations.

She was eighty-two by the time of her consultation at the unit, on a bleak October day. She came alone. She was elegantly dressed, with a striped silk shirt reminiscent of a Missoni design, and a carefully adjusted taupe scarf. She had a sharp face and a long nose. As she sat down, prompted by the neurologist, she said she was furious at what had happened to her after that laser operation for melanoma in her eye. She spoke of it as if it had happened the day before – even though the intervention had taken place three years previously. 'I lost my speech,' she said as she sat down, in response to the doctor's usual opening question, 'so, what is wrong?' She seemed at once outraged and mournful. Outside there was a strong wind, and the blinds hit the windows incessantly. The sky was overcast, a flat white over the 1970s buildings in the south of the hospital grounds. 'I was in a haze,' she went on. She meant she was in a haze after the laser operation. 'Anaesthesia lasts. I can't write, or see. I can't remember anything, it's a catastrophe. I used to have an elephant's memory. I can't speak properly, and I can't use the phone. I can't understand what I read because I don't see words as continuous.'

Her complaints were many. There were her hallucinations.

Hers were visual, not acoustic like Toussaint's. There were visits from the dead, illusions, sensations of things touching her. Every day, things around her transformed into other things. Inert objects became people, faces, arms. She was very lucid about the experience, which she described vividly. As she spoke, she suddenly pointed to an empty stool next to the doctor's chair, saying, 'Here, you see, it's a face, I see its eyes, they're blinking.' Unlike Toussaint, she understood these apparent transformations were not real. Her hallucinations had started a few years before, when she began seeing her dead brother, sundry children she didn't even know – and her husband, who she presumed was dead, though he had never been found, either dead or alive. 'They don't look for people in France. My husband disappeared but they didn't bother to look for him – we're a free country they say.' She was angry about that, too.

Then she said: 'I live on the top floor of a building. I see the whole city from there. I don't get much sleep. My husband had always been a calm man, but with the progression of the disease he'd become choleric.' Her quickened speech was full of non-sequiturs of this kind, though she often was at a loss for the right word, much to her annoyance. In the anamnesis, she had been described as always having had logorrhea – she simply talked too much, all the time, in a mode that was fast and tense. She also seemed to have some sort of persecution syndrome: she was the sort of person who complained to the police about whatever she could complain of – including what she saw as the police's own unwillingness to look for her husband. She fought with her family. There was a testimonial from her son, according to whom her mood, which had always been on the irritable side, had worsened: she had become excessively talkative, aggressive with everyone, so unbearable in fact that he suspected his demented father had fled the facility to avoid having to see her. By now, he barely spoke to her. And indeed her anger permeated the room.

Yet she had a dynamic mien that contrasted with that negative picture and her negative self-perception. She was unwell, she said. She needed help. And unlike some patients who entered unsure of whether they could trust the doctors, she seemed keen on the medical community. She rather endearingly called the neurologist whom she had met the day before 'my little angel'. Something about her, right there beneath her anger and anxiety, was much less off-putting than the family testimony and anamnesis had led one to believe. She was self-aware, self-possessed, and clearly intelligent. She had led a sophisticated life, and spoken four languages. So she was all the more frustrated by the difficulties she faced, embarrassed by her growing forgetfulness, by the words escaping her grasp ever more frequently – even though her linguistic fluency was in fact far better on neuropsychological tests, whose results were reported in the anamnesis, than her own evaluation of it. 'I lose track all the time,' she said. 'Can one get memory back? I'm not staying this way. I need help for the eye medicine. I'm alone. All noises frighten me. I see objects. If I hear a noise I know it's a person. It's hard to get help.'

Her eye operation had made things worse and enhanced her hallucinations: with the cataract in the other eye, by now she saw very little of her actual surroundings. She had other kinds of hallucinations as well, synaesthetic ones, where the boundaries between the senses were blurred – she had felt tree branches touching her once, a touch hallucination – though now she had no recollection of the experience, as if it had taken place in the netherworlds of her mind. She was socially isolated, and by all accounts her persecution syndrome had been getting worse over the past few years. She had trouble answering the questions that the neurologist asked her during her examination. Prompted to tell the tale of the Three Little Pigs, she meandered, got lost, gave up. She then returned to her anger with the 'awful' surgeon who had performed the laser eye operation, and who, she believed, had caused her incapacities – her loss of words, her difficulty in recognizing objects or writing numbers. 'Since the laser I've been floating. It was all white in there – I was lost. I hear things, to me they never say the truth. They lost my notes four times over here – you are all so disorganized! I told the secretary. I can organize you! Can I recuperate my good memory? I'm drugged, how can I be de-drugged? I get lost in my local supermarket.'

She had been staying at a friend's house because hers had become so disordered she couldn't recognize it. 'I thought someone had made a mess. I couldn't remember the name of my street. I don't like my house. If my husband were around it wouldn't be like that. There are packages everywhere.' When asked whether she had ever entertained negative thoughts such as ending it all, she admitted that, yes, she often thought of jumping out of her high window, up there on the eighteenth floor. 'I want to leave,' she said. 'I am fed up.' I had noticed that the doctors in the room never tiptoed around that question, impressive in their ability to lift the lid on suicidal ideation, straightforwardly calling it what it is and thus, perhaps, allowing the healing to begin. But she seemed to be holding on. She was at once chaotic and coherent, perplexed and confident still.

Then she told us: 'About a year ago, in the house my daughter built in Normandy, I was reading on the sofa. Then I saw my husband, who looked normal, not sick. "Can I sit?", he asked. I saw the sofa cushion move. It was all in colour. I was awake – it was not a dream.' She was patient and fluent as she spoke of her husband's sudden appearance.

'What did you make of it?' asked the doctor.

'"Oh, if only it could be true!" I said to myself. "I won't move." He sat down, I assure you. I was contented, it was a signal that he was not far. I'm not Catholic, I have no religion, this was not from God. I wanted to touch him. But there was nothing to touch. It never happened again. He never returned.'

'Do you think this was real, or imagined?'

'Oh, it was not imagined. My niece had a premonition that her mother would die, and she did, the next day. Two months I looked for my husband. Two months. They don't look for people, they say. Free country, my foot.'

She rambled some more. Everything was confused. But that appearance of her husband had been clear as the light of day.

Geraldine didn't want to leave the room when the time came for her to do so. She liked the attentive listeners who were sitting around the white table. 'You don't pity me, which is a good thing,' she said as she finally exited to be led back to her room. She was not well, and she knew it. Something of her layered, complex personality had emerged out of the pathological characterization that had been in her anamnesis, and I realized I wasn't sure what to make of her. I then reminded myself that there was nothing to make of her, clinically speaking: the point of her seeing the doctors in that hospital room was to find out what was wrong and how she could be helped. Her difficult character may indeed have been part of the pathology that needed unravelling, though this wasn't a given. I realized how quickly both social and emotional judgements have to be discarded, to make space for the subtle empathy without which the patient's suffering cannot be properly heard or understood.

Once Geraldine left the room, the neurologist who had examined her told us about Charles Bonnet Syndrome, or CBS. (He addressed in particular the medical students: their weekly presence ensured there was a didactic aspect to these sessions, which helped me acquire a rudimentary education in the basics of neurology.) Geraldine's hallucinations, he explained – those that we witnessed her having during the examination – were an example of it, at least in part, because her eyesight was so bad. The syndrome was named after the eighteenth-century,

Swiss-born, French naturalist Charles Bonnet, a lawyer by profession who, like a number of his contemporaries in that age of scientific revolution, was a keen entomologist and botanist.[2]

Bonnet studied many aspects of the natural world, and became a member of scientific societies throughout Europe.[3] But once his eyesight started deteriorating, microscopic observation became impossible, and he started developing broader theories regarding human psychology, as well as participating in the philosophical debates of his day, adopting the notion advanced by John Locke that all knowledge arises from sense-experience.[4] He took note, for example, of what his eighty-seven-year-old grandfather, Charles Lullin, was undergoing. Partially blind from cataracts, Lullin had begun having hallucinations of extraordinary sophistication and Bonnet himself later experienced the same thing. He reported and discussed his grandfather's experience in an essay published in 1760,[5] and Oliver Sacks, in his book on hallucinations, republished a summary of Lullin's own account. During a visit by his grand-daughters one day, Lullin saw young men dressed in red and grey cloaks, wearing silver-trimmed hats. Then the figures dissolved as mysteriously as they had appeared. The visions, on this and on other occasions, were often rather grand, but also odd, involving women with boxes on their heads, giant carriages, a floating handkerchief, or a miniature scaffold in his own living room, encountered after he had seen a real, normal-sized one while walking through town earlier that day.[6]

The syndrome Bonnet described, which is also called 'visual release hallucinations', is usually specific to people who have lost all or part of their visual faculty, due to opthalmological disorders.[7] Although understanding of the workings of the brain was rudimentary at this point, Bonnet correctly surmised that, in the absence of an external stimulus, the visions had to come from cerebral activity in visual areas of the brain,

triggering, he thought, visual memories. He saw it as a confusion of 'vision and reality'. Brain imaging has indeed shown
that the same areas of the brain are activated in the perception
of, say, a face, and in the hallucination of a face – though not
when one is imagining a face. In other words, such hallucinations are closer to perception than to imagination.[8]

I am not old yet, and have reasonably good eyesight. But
in the early 2000s, I witnessed from up close *what it is like* to
have such strange visions. Late in her long life, an elderly
friend, the entomologist and zoologist Miriam Rothschild,
became afflicted with exactly this syndrome. It would appear
most frequently in the evening – a characteristic of the
syndrome – then subside. And it so happens that she too was
a naturalist and entomologist, like Bonnet.[9] I will never know
whether she knew that her visions bore the clinical name of
a man whose work she must have been familiar with: I didn't
know enough at the time to ask her, having never heard of
either him, or the syndrome.

Like many children of her class, gender, and generation, she
had been brought up by nannies and educated by tutors at
home. She became a highly accomplished scientist, eventually
running experiments around the world, and authoring or
co-authoring many scientific papers, books and memoirs. She
was a forceful presence and something of an eccentric, endowed
with a lively, passionate mind, high energy, a great sense of
humour about the absurdities of human life, and a deep love
of poetry and literature. Despite her age, I thought of her as
a close friend, and felt lucky I could. Her conversation roamed
far and wide. She had a prodigious memory that enabled her
to tell mesmerizing stories about the natural world, recite
poetry, tell the life stories of her many acquaintances, friends
and lovers, and recall whole dialogues with everyone she had
ever met. She was dedicated to science, and to issues of nature
conservation – like her father who had created the nature

reserve where she lived, and where I visited her about once a month over the dozen or so years I lived in London.

She lost her senses one by one, all except touch. First taste, devastating for anyone who loves to eat, as she did – especially chocolate, a passion we shared. (My mother loves chocolate too, and her loss of taste luckily doesn't seem to include chocolate.) Then hearing, to some extent. Last, and most debilitatingly for her, sight. Her extraordinary mental faculties remained intact. One early spring evening, we were finishing dinner at the dining-room table, just she and I. Dusk was settling over the garden outside the tall windows. We hadn't switched on the lights yet. Our conversation had turned wistful, even melancholy, as it often did by the end of meals, and by the end of her life – she would die a few years later, aged ninety-six. Suddenly, she said, 'Oh look, all those people in elegant dresses walking down the hill there. This must be Tring! And look at those horses. There's a carriage, too.' (She was old enough to have seen horses and carriages in her childhood; Tring was the estate where she had grown up.)

I was astounded. She wasn't. She knew perfectly well what was happening. She lived in a penumbra and these bright visions became a regular occurrence – though she did not name them as anything other than visions. Bonnet hallucinations are 'critiqued', meaning that they are not delusions: one is aware that they are hallucinations. But they can be impressive all the same. They turned bleaker when we got up from the table and started traversing the darkened living room: the furniture abruptly turned into piles of stone and bricks, obstacles I had to help her circumnavigate. Now she grew distressed. She said it all looked horrible. She asked me to accompany her to her bedroom – she was in a wheelchair, as she had been for over a decade, because of back issues. Thankfully the visions had vanished and she regained her composure by the time we reached her room. She turned on the light, and bade me goodnight.

Geraldine's hallucinations were of the Charles Bonnet type, then. They were caused, at least in part, by the near-blindness that had also afflicted my friend Miriam. In the total or almost total absence of sight, a whole world was re-constructed, that was at once 'out there' and not. In the absence of visual stimuli, the brain produces complex images, woven into memory as were the sounds in the AVH Toussaint had experienced. Like AVH, CBS provides evidence that the brain *generates* visual or (in the case of AVH) auditory representations, regardless of any input from the outside world. One could say that, in reaction to the loss of such input, the brain overcompensates, somewhat as in the phenomenon of phantom limbs. And the overcompensation could be understood as the homeostatic regulation of neurons that usually process external input. In the absence of exteroceptive input (that our senses – in this case, eyes – process from the outside world), these neuronal circuits recruit imagery out of memory traces, and out of interoceptive signals from the body itself. And interoception affects proprioception – the sense we have of our dynamic, musculoskeletal body in space (how, for example, I know where my arm is when I wake up in the dark), and the ability to move around in space.[10]

Miriam's experience of CBS hallucinations, on this reading, would have been an embodied memory, affecting her whole body, and her proprioceptive sense. Perhaps it was that the visions occupied her peripersonal space – the space around her body – as so many obstacles, menacing her free movement and her sense of agency within the room she otherwise knew so well, transforming her bodily self-consciousness, and all the embodied memory that was part of it.[11] Hence the horse and carriages that emerged in the park outside the living-room windows from the depths of her early life. Our body carries our life's memories, registered in a multimodal palimpsest that constitutes who we are at any given point in time. When one sense modality is disrupted, damaged, or destroyed, our embodied sense of self within the present moment is affected. At any rate, this is how, some twenty years later, I attempt to understand what my friend may have experienced on that evening – and perhaps many times until she died.

Geraldine had similar CBS hallucinations. But beyond those, her experience differed widely from my friend's. Notably, the perceptual misjudgment that had led her to see her vanished husband sitting on the sofa did not seem to partake of CBS. Brain imaging had showed a hypometabolism – a lowered processing of glucose, which indicates less energy use, and thus less activity – in the primary visual cortex, which is located in the occipital lobe. This meant that her failing eyesight was not only due to her retinal deterioration. It must have been also due to a neurological issue, since in CBS there is no hypometabolism in the visual cortex, which remains active as it generates imagery.

That neurological issue, surmised the doctors, could therefore be connected to her other symptoms, which included her incoherent speech – the verbal paraphrasia and circumlocutions – her losing track of narratives and ideas, her distractability, the reported mess in her house, and the fact that her statements were not socially adapted. Moreover, she exhibited what neuropsychologists call 'perseveration' – repetition of a word or gesture once the stimulus for it has ceased, and the inability to switch tasks or change tack, indicative of a dysfunction in the ability to control automatic behaviour in the light of new information. All of these elements, the doctors agreed, were connected. They pointed to a 'dysexecutive syndrome', that disorder of the executive syndrome we have met before, generally associated with the prefrontal lobe, and involved in our putting ideas together, understanding cues and controlling our impulses. Not mentioned in this clinical setting was that this does not mean the executive has a 'supervisory' function. There is no *homunculus* sitting on our frontal lobe overlooking our actions.[12] The functions of the prefrontal cortex are highly integrated with other brain areas, processing states of arousal and homeostatic regulation according to intentions and goals that partake of emotional, interoceptive cues.[13] One cannot reduce mental functions to discrete brain areas any more than one can reduce a person to just the brain.

Yet inevitably the discussion was focused on Geraldine's brain. We had left the realm of her messed-up life on the high floor of her building from which she saw the whole city, for a somewhat abstract, detached detective world, a whodunnit of cerebral pathology. There was suspense, there were clinical minds at work to put together the pieces of the puzzle into a diagnostic portrait that would be in the likeness of Geraldine. It was significant, thought the neurologists, that she had believed her husband's appearance to be real. She did not doubt that, somehow, he had appeared to her – not in flesh and blood exactly, since she had not been able to touch him, but as the person he had been before he had become ill. When she had recounted the episode, she had been unable to jump to a rational conclusion about it. The doctors surmised that her deluded belief, which also may have reflected a deep wish (or a worry) could be either an aspect of the dysexecutive syndrome, or of a pathology involving the posterior lobe. Those were two very different possibilities. But the fact that she had not thought herself mad, and that in the retelling of the episode she did not rationally revise her interpretation, indicated that it was more likely her prefrontal lobe was affected.

Together with the dysexecutive symptoms, they said, the delusional hallucination could perhaps be indicative of a neuro-degenerative disease called Lewy Body Dementia, or LBD.[14] The illness evolves slowly, progressively affecting various cognitive, emotional, and motor functions, in many areas of the brain. This is also the case with Alzheimer's Disease, or AD, although LBD patients are not necessarily anosognosic and, on the contrary, can be painfully aware of their condition. Both are so-called 'proteinopathies' – illnesses where proteins essential in complex ways to brain function go rogue, as it were.[15] Very little is understood about the why and how of these neurodegenerative diseases, despite their prevalence amongst the general, particularly the aging, population, and the huge financial resources that are devoted to research related to them. My mother is just one of many millions of people struck with one of these terrible afflictions. Geraldine may well be another.

One of the neurologists told us of a LBD patient who would wake in the middle of the night, telling his wife that he saw someone on the outside patio with a flashlight looking in. He also saw people outside the bedroom window – it is quite typical for LBD hallucinations to involve figures, including small people, as if seen through glass. He wasn't disturbed by these visions any more than if they had been a dream. The visual association areas in the visual cortex are activated in these occurrences just as they are with ordinary visual perception. The brain creates the visual experience as it does in dreams – it is a dream-like phenomenon that occurs while awake. At that stage of the disease, he would ask during the day, 'who is that old woman dancing in that elegant green outfit, who are all these other people who have arrived and won't leave?' The hallucination diminished with social interaction. But he wondered how he could be sure that what he saw was not actually there, as he was told.

Geraldine seemed to have experienced something similar. Her husband had arrived as a dream of sorts, vivid and embodied enough so that the effect lingered and became a part of her remembered reality – or so one could interpret her certainty about the reality of his appearance. Her anger and outrage at the inability of the authorities to find him may have played a part in the tenor and emotional valence – the emotional character – of that vision, too. At any rate, LBD was not yet a certain diagnosis, though it was likely. Other tests had to be done to confirm what ailment was afflicting her brain. A scintigraphy – an imaging technique that uses a radioactive tracer – had been performed already, which showed that her prefrontal cortex was in surprisingly good shape. This result excluded another degenerative disorder called Fronto-Temporal Dementia (FTD), characterized by a loss of impulse control, inhibition, judgement, empathy, and so on, due to damage to the frontotemporal lobe. The doctors determined that, in order to fix a diagnosis, more imaging was needed, including a DaTscan to measure her dopamine levels, a reduced level of which was indicative of LBD.[16] She also needed a lumbar puncture (or LP) to test the cerebrospinal fluid for the presence of proteins that would attest to Alzheimer's disease. An abnormal DaTscan and normal LP would probably signal Lewy Body Dementia. The opposite would point to Alzheimer's. The former was more likely, thought the neurologists, because of the nature of her hallucinations, including her synaesthetic ones, which seemed to take place just as she was waking from REM sleep. Her sleeping difficulties were typical of LBD: the sleep/wake cycle is eroded in the course of the disease, though that is also the case in other dementias.[17] And she needed some form of home care. In any case, it was inevitable that the disease would spread, and undermine her normal functioning, from memory and language to sleep, smell, and movement, increasingly affecting her emotions.

One may wonder what is the point of pinpointing exactly the nature of an ailment doctors can do so little about, besides prescribe anxiety-reducing drugs if they are needed. But a doctor's job is to understand and offer whatever help is available. We had seen Geraldine as the neurodegenerative process had begun. She was still in character, and justifiably furious: her life was marked by a severe loss – that of her husband, first to AD, then to the geographical unknown. The psychiatrist in the room said at one point that 'one hallucinates one's desires.' Indeed if hallucinations are midway between dreams and perceptions, then they are more potent than imagination. They can provide fulfillment, as the apparition of her husband did in Geraldine's case. What the police were unable to deliver, her own mind did. She held on to that one instance as to a revelatory moment. But to the medical eye, that instance was a symptom of a disease that eventually was going to take much more away from her.

It was to be hoped that Geraldine would find the support and care she needed from here on. The exact nature of her dementia might not matter in the end. Most people who accompany a member of their family on the downward path of neuro-degeneration do not care so much about what the name of that path might be. I don't either. But dementias, and the nature of their course, do vary hugely, in both their symptoms and in how aware the patient is of the affliction. Whether they manifest in memory or behavioural issues, the dementias may not even be one kind of disease, as some neurologists believe. The clinical types rarely match the textbook pathology they are supposed to correspond to. Pathologies are many and combine in dozens of ways – and there can be 'co-morbidities', too, a combination of many illnesses within one organism. The neurological canon has distinct symptomatologies, but the labels are tenuous. One neurologist at the hospital argued that the broad term 'neurodegeneration' may eventually be abandoned in favour of that of 'proteinopathy', given that such illnesses share the characteristic of proteins gone rogue. We are at the mercy of the proteins that bind us. They can become unbound, and when they do our lives and layers unwind.

It is all fascinating, in its way. In fact the only redeeming aspect of an illness may be its scientific interest, if one is interested in such matters, from the molecular level up: how protein tangles affect dopaminergic systems and the bases of consciousness, while language remains, and the 'I' remains too. I can't help being fascinated even as my mother's inner world gradually contracts – I feel able to step away from the personal experience, to take a distance from the baffling reality and my inexpressible emotions. These very pages emerge out of the to and fro between the subjective and the objective, the experience and the contemplation, mine as well as that of others. I am fascinated by our general capacity for metacognition, after all. And grateful to the scientists and clinicians. My father died of a rare cancer and at the worst of times was buoyed up by his interest in his own case. He enjoyed his exchanges with the nurses and doctors, and they loved this intensely interested patient. His mental faculties, as was the case with Miriam – who had been his friend long before my birth – were intact until his last breath. He was fully aware. He even celebrated his eighty-first birthday the day before he died. The strangeness of dementia is that while mental faculties decline, and awareness ultimately vanishes, it doesn't look like an illness: aside from an insecure gait, my mother's bodily health is fairly solid so far, and she is in her late eighties. She takes no medication. And she looks at least ten years younger than her age.

When faced with this unwinding of a person one is close to, one can only observe, accept the ride, be present, help, and seek help. And laugh, too. My mother luckily does not have the signs of LBD – she has no hallucinations, for instance. We are only conjecturing that she has AD, since we have decided not to test for its biomarkers: it makes little sense to subject her to an invasive lumbar puncture, given how little one can do to help in any case, and given that, whatever it is she has, it is making her serene. It is as if this particular proteinopathy, to call it that, were bringing out the most life-loving, giving, affectionate, exuberant, humorous and gracious aspects of her personality, enhancing it. In this sense, her anosognosia is a blessing.[18] Her relation to people is still emotionally full. It is just devoid of coherent references, and the verbal exchanges that have replaced conversation have become surreal – hilariously so, sometimes. It helps that they are peppered with those one-liners I write down. 'Where are the children?' I asked the other day when we all visited her, and suddenly they could be neither seen nor heard from the living room where we were sitting. 'They're being brainwashed,' she responded, and then laughed.

She knows who she is, still, and she knows who I am. She still tells me how to wear my unruly curly hair – and when she does, it is as if nothing had changed. As long as she can criticize my hair, the mother I knew still exists. The mother who, many years ago, laughed heartily with me in shared self-recognition at a *New Yorker* cartoon in which a mother and daughter are browsing in a bookstore, and while the mother looks at the 'Biography' section, the daughter, standing at the nearby 'Criticism' section, tells her, 'Look, Mother, this section should interest you.' The hair moments are little specks of light within her growing penumbra. But she no longer gets the cartoon. The unravelling goes on. She is disoriented in time and space, unable to hold on to facts – a 'dysexecutive syndrome' in full play. She does not know where she is within her embodied temporality, which explains why she depends on her carers to attend to her personal hygiene. Her internal schedule is off-kilter: she awakes in the middle of the night believing it is morning, her circadian clock and embodied sense of time as distorted as the haunting clocks in those Dalì paintings that used to terrify me when I was small. (Circadian disturbances are typical of many dementias, not just LBD – which is why her waking up in the middle of the night in London was a portent.)[19] When, as I re-ordered my wardrobe to meet the spring, I found a top she had bought for me a few years ago, it occurred to me that I will never receive another gift from her. She can no longer go shopping and can't remember she ever did. She cannot grasp where she is in the space and time of the world, of her life, of her memories, of others.

And it is not just cartoons we no longer can laugh at together. She also no longer remembers what she likes. I can no longer share articles and books with her, nor show her my work as I always used to, and as I did one last time, on that last Eurostar ride, which she will have forgotten by now. The news of the historic Covid-19 pandemic during which I write these lines somewhat pierces through to her awareness, but not quite. ('Mummy half the planet is confined!' 'Well, they won't confine me!') My younger son says memory is a labyrinth in which she has got lost. References are diminishing fast. The humorous wordplay cannot hide that the world has become, from her perspective, a place of chaos – it may even reveal the chaos. 'I can't see the letters but I saw the words,' she quipped recently. The verbal agility sometimes translates into an unconscious awareness. 'I'm so ok I can't stand it.' I don't know what the world looks like for her – in contrast to my vivid sense of what Miriam's dimmed dining room looked like to her when she had the Bonnet hallucinations, all those years ago. Teapots go on the hob, pyjamas are buttoned across the dressy shirt – all part of what is called 'ideational apraxia', the inability to identify the tasks associated with objects. She is rarely hungry and forgets to drink, her interoceptive signalling as off-kilter as her inner clock.[20] All dementias ultimately distort agency, the engrammed self, the body-in-the-world, the time in this world.

Many more people live longer lives today, so the rate of dementias of all sorts has gone up.[21] But dementia is no new story. Shakespeare, in *The Winter's Tale*, has Polixenes ask Florizel:

> Is not your father grown incapable
> Of reasonable affairs? is he not stupid
> With age and alt'ring rheums? can he speak? hear?
> Know man from man? dispute his own estate?
> Lies he not bed-rid? and again does nothing
> But what he did being childish?[22]

The correlation of age with mental decline has always been observed, and understood as a natural, though not necessarily inevitable occurrence. Galen, the influential Roman second-century physician, found that the brains of older animals were smaller than those of younger ones, assuming from those smaller brains that the corresponding minds were less nimble. And he described what he called 'morosis' as the 'extreme debility' that, in old age, leads to symptoms of massive memory loss.[23] The Hippocratic system of the four humours that he inherited and developed associated old age with the element of earth, its qualities cold and dry, and the corresponding humour of black bile, or melancholy.[24] Imagine a cold, dry brain. Look at the melancholy of aging.

It remains difficult to separate the notion of mental decline from that of life's decline. We are impressed by elderly people whose minds are intact, because we expect that the wrinkles on the skin will correspond to rumples in the brain. Florizel's response to Polixenes is:

> No, good sir;
> He has his health and ampler strength indeed
> Than most have of his age.

The 'most' is not a precise term, but it indicates how much we expect age to weigh down on health. The question of when 'age' begins to weigh varies, however – from person to person, and according to families, classes, cultures, population groups.[25]

Some people, such as my father, and Miriam, do not age in their minds, but acquire a host of ailments in their bodies – including the various cancers our cells are so alarmingly capable of turning into. 'The machine is breaking down,' one may hear from many an older person beset with debilitating arthritis and deafness, say. The language of dualism re-appears in these cases. Others, such as my mother, will suffer neurological damage, while the rest of the body remains mostly intact. In all these cases, the reality of the self seems oddly dual, the aging process as if on two separate speeds, neurons obeying one temporal order, and the cells in the rest of the body another. But the person is never just one or the other. Our emotive states modulate our immune system and the inflammatory processes that can produce illnesses.

During the eighteen months over which I witnessed the sessions, I saw quite a few people come into that room with what turned out to be incipient neurodegenerative diseases. In most cases they were still fully themselves, right on the brink of the loss of any imagined future, and of the slow, irreversible fading of much of their past. Their condition was rarely easy to determine through clinical examination alone. There are a myriad of signs that a doctor must attend to in order to understand the patient in the context of their life history. For instance, it is hard to tease out if a depression signals the arrival of a dementia, or is caused by it. Technology helps, especially given the advances in neuroimaging,[26] but the clinic always precedes it: the maps that brain imaging provide can help answer questions, but the questions must first be formulated. They are mute without an expert reader and the clinical observation of the fragilities and labilities of each patient. Each time, I saw how crucial it was for the doctor never to presume before looking and listening, testing hand-clapping, walking, grasping. Diagnosis takes place in that space between what we understand and what we don't. The diagnostic process in the case of Geraldine was focused on what could be understood about the neuropathological symptoms. Her complex personality, so much harder to make out, was not part of the discussion. What was examined in that room was how an illness wound itself into the life and character of a person.

Yet as I have been learning during these days of decline in my mother's life, the pathology is not the whole story of that person – not unless and until it reaches the last, gruesomely vegetative stage. It determines the logistics of a life, but the core self does remain, even as the autobiographical self disperses progressively[27] – to adopt the distinction formulated by Antonio Damasio, who also describes how Alzheimer's disease erodes 'the bedrock of autobiographical memory', how he saw neurons in areas key to its functioning 'turned into tombstones'.[28] So much is lost – neurons dying as time ticks and even as I type – but for now my mother's hand feels the same on my hand or face as it did when I was a child. The voice. The pressure, temperature, feel of the skin. The way she taps on one part of my cheek. That level of embodied, intimate personhood has not changed a bit. One could only hope that Geraldine's son would take her by the hand too. That he would get over his understandable anger with her and forgive her anger in turn – relent, accept the ride, and give her respite from the solitude that had been plaguing her since her husband disappeared after his own unravelling had begun.

6

Guilty as Charged

Je suis le Ténébreux, – le Veuf, – l'Inconsolé,
Le Prince d'Aquitaine à la Tour abolie:
Ma seule Etoile est morte, – et mon luth
    constellé
Porte le Soleil noir de la Mélancolie.

Gérard de Nerval,
from 'El Desdichado', in *Les Chimères* (1854)

My mother still has her inner world, but it no longer corresponds to the world shared by most people who go about ordinary lives, work, have families, take care of their homes, plan the dinner, discuss the news, read books, tweet their opinions, go on holiday, and take photographs. Still, it is hers, inalienably so. A recurring theme in her world is the need to get hold of people by telephone: when I want to speak to her carer, who may even be in the same room, she says she will hang up now so she can telephone her. A trace of her anxiety about reaching people remains, along with her warm sociability. And she still assumes that sociability about herself: a measure of self-knowledge therefore lives on, connected to her strong affect rather than to the devastated narrative, autobiographical memory. There is such a thing as 'cognitive reserve', and it is on display here – the legacy of a lifetime of reading, writing, and learning – expressed in her strong connections to people as well as in her agile verbal puns.[1] 'I'm full of power and pointlessness,' she said once. She may remain in this state for a while, full of power and pointlessness, or her power may deteriorate fast, to the point of life becoming pointless. We cannot predict. No one course of illness is like another.

But it occurs to me at times, after I finish a video chat with her and, then, with some relief, shunt it all to the side of a busy day and attend to my life, that the assumption of normality can be constraining. It is the equivalent of health, and health is never a guaranteed good. It is humbling, to say the least, to remember that all we take for granted as the basis of a cogent, livable life, can disintegrate. We live instead in a rather arrogant world of executive function and executive diaries, with little space for the dysexecutive. Pathology is off the charts – a nasty parenthesis, the hospital and hospice space, the business of the medical profession. Yet preserving space for the literally extra-ordinary may be another way of looking at a disrupted mind, in a way that preserves the richness of a lived life even while ordinary cognition is impaired. The patients I saw were all somewhere between the ordinary and the extra-ordinary, and their difficulties manifested again and again how subtle is the passage from normality to pathology, how invisible, often, is the break-off point beyond which one can become lost to the world. Complex mechanisms are at work in ensuring a correspondence between self-perception and the perception of oneself by others. In the case of my mother, that correspondence no longer exists. It is a disturbing asymmetry. That is the nature of anosognosia: you may feel and know yourself as normal, but actually something is terribly wrong with you. You can't see it – but I can.

Anosognosia takes as many forms as self-knowledge. We are always within a blind spot, whose size varies, like the eye's pupil. Sometimes the light comes in, but sometimes the darkness takes over. The clinician must try to understand where a person is within the darkness – taking a step into the dysexecutive realm, looking at normality from that side, rather than at pathology from the end of normality. It is a deeply empathic movement. I realize now, as I struggle to construct a new relationship with my mother, how hard it is to achieve, and to preserve communication within (or despite) the asymmetry. Such empathy was particularly hard to achieve in the case of a memorable patient I shall call Eric, whose consultation was so unexpectedly extreme that I was compelled to write about him in the present tense.

Eric is terribly thin, bespectacled, and has a neat three-day beard. He wears a striped polo shirt. We learn from the anamnesis that he was diagnosed with Parkinson's Disease a few years ago, in his early sixties. And for a long time, since his early twenties, he has known the ups and downs of bipolar disorder: depression, followed by hypomania, and back again. It took years for the disorder to be diagnosed. When Eric walks into the room, he has been depressed for about six months this time round. He has been seeing a psychiatrist, though the episode has been worsening. He takes many medications, but they don't seem to be helping his mood. His judgement is clouded. He is slow: he has what neurologists call bradykinesia, those slow movements characteristic of Parkinson's.[2]

Eric also feels terribly guilty, according to the anamnesis, and is afflicted by a form of delirium whose nature and origin are not clear, and which began before he went on the medications. He sees the world as a dangerous place, and himself as having done it infinite harm. He may have some form of psychosis, but the delirium may also be an aspect of his Parkinson's. He is on a low dose of Levodopa, or L-Dopa,[3] which Oliver Sacks made famous in his *Awakenings*, and where he described its miraculous effects on patients affected with sleeping sickness.⁴ When Eric comes in, he just stands there, his gaze lost in space, his whole body rigid, arms straight along the body. He is entirely silent. He seems not to care at all about anything that is happening around him. He gazes at us as upon abject objects. His anamnesis, an odd combination of life history and pharmacological compendium, revealed that he had wanted to take religious orders, but it never happened. He wanted to teach theology, but only found a job at a packing company. Even there, though, he held on to his higher aspirations, and tried to look high up, every day. His voice only makes sense, it seems, when it is directed at the heavens.

When the neurologist asks Eric how he feels, he says nothing. He is not looking at the doctors, or at anyone around the table. The neurologist explains, as he always does, that all these people are doctors, whose purpose is to work out what is wrong and what can be done to help. In a tiny voice, Eric says, 'Yes, it makes quite an impression to be in front of all these people.' The doctor asks a few more standard questions. Eric barely responds, though he does register them. Then, in that same windless, barely audible voice, as if it were being effortfully squeezed out of a tight space, he declares: 'I don't deserve the trust of others. I've accepted that I didn't accept the things that occur in life. I no longer deserve to live. I didn't used to think that. Now I do.'

The examination is a painful struggle. Both neurologists attempt to extricate something more out of this man. It is hard for them to know how to ask the patient about what they need to know, to extract some sort of usable data from his experience. Eric knows he is depressed, that much he acknowledges. And he sleeps badly. 'I'm not well at all, this time round.' The psychiatrist attempts to contextualize the dark pit in which Eric stands, explaining to him what people typically feel when they're depressed. Eric says he also sometimes senses people want to harm him. And he hears voices, addressed to him

– some positive, some negative. 'My mind is wobbly.' He meanders. 'Do you think this hospital stay will help you?' asks the psychiatrist. '. . . A little' is the answer, long in coming. 'Do you think you'll get over it?' Long seconds, then: 'I have hope.' The medications are helping a little – for the motor issues associated with Parkinson's. 'And for the head?' asks the doctor. No response.

I think again as he sits, trapped within his terrible silence, facing people who are clearly functioning well, driven, healthy: there is the person, then the patient, then the brain. To what extent am I not my brain, if any glitch in that organ has an effect on how I sense, move, stand, think, remember, perceive, feel, eat, sleep, control thoughts and feelings? What aspect of myself and life does it not affect? And conversely, what aspects of our lives are not dependent on the brain's smooth functioning? Eric's guilt is generated from within himself. He is the one to feel it, and he feels isolated by it. And yet guilt is a *social* emotion, and all social emotions are shared between individuals: they are not 'in' the brain, even though we use our brains to process them. What is Eric guilty about? Why is he silent? Why aren't we all silent? The person, then the patient, then the brain. Or is it the other way round?

Some information does come out. He is tired. He has low energy, though it can be variable. His appetite is not very good: he has lost a lot of weight – 18 kg. He is a wisp of a man. He is almost nothing. It occurs to me he is like Kafka's hunger artist who has nearly departed his body. He is the incarnation of a negative thought, what remains after a 'melancholic hurricane', as the psychiatrist calls it. The silence continues. The neurologist tries again. 'When you don't answer, why is this? Empty mind? Many things in mind? Hard to concentrate? When one asks you a question, does it trigger a thought that takes you elsewhere?' The questions aim at finding out how wobbly his thought process really is. 'It happens' is the slow, barely audible reply. Eric seems to want to hold on to the feeling of knowing better than the doctor. But the doctor knows a lot, too.

The other neurologist tries a different tack, more emotionally direct and explicit, more authoritative: 'There are things you said that sound terrible,' he says. 'That you don't deserve to live, or don't deserve the trust of people. It must be heavy to bear. If one doesn't deserve to live, one must have done terrible things. Have you done terrible things? We're not here to judge you. What have you done to deserve this? Have you done anything to deserve punishment? . . . You don't answer because it's too terrible, or is it none of my business? Have you killed someone? . . . Have you told yourself, "I'd rather die?" . . . Look at me! What do you think of what I'm saying? I say this to help you.' Silence. 'You want to go back to your room?' A soft, but clear, 'No.' 'You seem to feel menaced, in a den of lions.' It is time to leave. He gets up. He doesn't shake anyone's hand. But then he freezes – he will not budge. And it isn't a Parkinsonian freezing. He simply does not want to leave the room. Two of the junior doctors have to force him out.

Once he has left, the discussion begins. Eric is very slowed down, deeply reticent, depressed, and dissociated. He has lost touch with feelings of hunger – this is why he has become so terribly thin. His mood is fluctuating. It is a case of catatonic negativism, says the psychiatrist, a delirium where all questions are perceived as persecution. Or a schizoaffective disorder – a fairly rare disorder in which the delusional symptoms akin to those in schizophrenia are combined with the extreme swings between mania and depression typical of bipolar disorder.[5] It could also be an iatrogenic phenomenon, that is, one brought on by the medication.[6] Or, suggests one of the neurologists, a cortical illness, such as cortico-basal degeneration – CBD – which affects the cortex and the basal ganglia deep in the brain, the symptoms of which include many of those typical of Parkinson's, such as slow movements, stiffness, tremors, and so on.[7] The neuropsychological tests he has undergone, however, do not indicate any cortical degradation. Eric does have Parkinson's, that much is certain. And he also has psychosis, undoubtedly.

Suddenly a loud knock on the door interrupts the proceedings. It is Eric. He wants to return. He has a statement to make. He walks back in. He now stands before us all, hands on table, as before a tribunal. There is another long silence. Then he speaks. 'I came in to ask for forgiveness for not having been up to what was expected of me. I tried to be, and thought I could go it alone. But I was wrong. I looked to the superior life. I failed.' He stops. Looks at all of us, one by one. There is a megalomaniac grandiosity here – the self-aggrandizing that can be associated with a number of psychiatric conditions. He is no longer so slowed down. The spectacle is compelling – a *coup de théâtre*. The speech seems to go on for a long time, though it only lasts two or three minutes. By the end, he thunders before the holy jury we have become: 'I request that all men forgive me!' And now he leaves, of his own volition. The trial is over. Guilty as charged.

It is hard to know what is going on in Eric's psyche: he has chosen to hide, from us if not from himself. It is significant, say the doctors, that Eric was only able to speak up after an hour of probing, triggering, and questioning: he seems to have little access to his own thoughts though he is not confused in any way. But it is unusual for a patient to return to the room after having been dismissed. It is as if he had to think through the scene, the possibilities, and his own beliefs and history before finally opening his mouth, entirely on his own terms, because answering questions in any other way would be beyond the pale for him. What he wants is a stage for a monologue. Eric is at the very far end of what one can recognize as ordinary experience. He is so wrapped up in despair that one wants to exclude him from the sphere of normality, precisely because it feels abhorrent to recognize anything normal in these extreme emotions. And yet, psychosis is a human, an all too human, experience. Guilt and grandiosity are typical symptoms of it, it would seem: inflated emotions in which the self is distorted, at once bloated and non-existent, as if the homeostatic mechanisms that govern its survival within the world had gone awry.[8] Here again the question arises of what has happened to the self whose mode of expression has become so tortured – so out of synch with the world and with social normality.

In the current *DSM 5*, psychosis is 'defined by abnormalities in one or more of the following five domains: delusions, hallucinations, disorganized thinking (speech), grossly disorganized or abnormal motor behavior (including catatonia), and negative symptoms'.[9] But the very nature of psychosis remains opaque, for reasons that run parallel to the historical separation of neurology from psychiatry and that correspond to the rationale that initially justified this separation. With the early twentieth-century detachment of psychiatry, which dealt with various forms of mental distress, from neurology, which dealt with locatable brain lesions, psychosis – the old 'vesania' of Pinel – fell under the purview of psychiatry. Where the object of neurology is the potentially visible, biological signature of disease, that of psychiatry is the invisible subjective state rooted in a self with its history. And so the status of the ailments in the ambit of psychiatry is inevitably amphibian: they are midway between biochemistry and the psyche. They overlap with the neurotic knots that psychoanalysis and all psychotherapies treat as well, and which tend not to consider biological data – while, in turn, psychiatry today is primarily biological in its approach, rather than rooted in a relational dialogue with psychoanalysis and its cognates. Freud's first calling, after all, was neurology, and he always conceived of the interpretative, semiotic, analytical, associative, archaeological method that became psychoanalysis as being complementary to psychiatry, not in opposition to it.[10]

Still, the psychoanalysis Freud founded, based as it was on inner narrative, diverged from the biological approach to mental illness that his contemporaries favoured, in particular the German psychiatrist Emil Kraepelin – whose classification of mental disorders persists today within psychiatry.[11] But it was a pupil of Kraepelin, the Swiss psychiatrist Eugen Bleuler, a crucial collaborator of Freud's, who was key to the transition from focusing on pathologies of the brain to crises of the psyche. Via his observations of patients over a dozen years, Bleuler focused on the complex psyche and inner workings of these patients, reconfiguring the understanding of what Kraepelin had called 'dementia praecox', and injecting a decidedly psychological perspective into the latter's organic approach.[12] This 'dementia praecox' broadly corresponds to what today we call schizophrenia, though this in turn was an appellation coined in 1891 by Arnold Pick (after whom is named Pick Disease, a specific form of fronto-temporal dementia, or FTD). Kraepelin eventually grouped the various versions of it that his predecessors had described into a 'uniform morbid process' for which he saw little chance of cure: these morbid processes were neurodegenerative ailments, *separate* from what he termed manic-depressive psychosis.[13]

The very notion that the pattern a disease takes could consist of a changing, progressing set of symptoms suggests that the name of a disease does not necessarily designate its symptoms, nor whatever proximal or immediate causes may be known or imagined. Naming any ailment begs questions about the assumptions being made regarding its nature. Psychosis is not a neurological disorder insofar as it is not 'located' in a specific area of the brain (as is a neurodegenerative disorder), no more than a personal history is either. Yet it has an organic dimension – all mental events do, and early psychiatry had originally been closely linked with neurology for that reason. Psychosis involves biochemical disturbances, as well as neurological dysfunctions.[14] Today, psychiatry treats mental illness with an arsenal of drugs targeting the receptors of neurotransmitters – and its patients tend to carry baggage that consists not only of their lives and psyches, but also of a pharmaceutical history that can be just as heavy. Eric is under many chemically calibrated medications whose names roll off the tongues of doctors as if they were old acquaintances, some of them intimate though sometimes troublesome friends. I found over the months I attended the clinic that many patients, and their families, made friends with those medications in a similar fashion, especially if they had been taking them for a long time. They were habituated to these little pills and expected their molecular charge, akin to drone-carried bombs that could cause unplanned ravage in their target's vicinity. I was often surprised at how many medications a person could be made to take in a day. Pharmacology is an important part of a doctor's medical knowledge, a crucial prop – for better and for worse – at the service of our complex cerebral chemistry.

A medication that acts upon neurophysiology can induce, augment, suppress, or transform the physiology underlying an emotional state. Yet chemistry and the modulations of neurotransmitters, however central in determining how we feel, are not the sole component in the dynamics of psychic life. Feelings, for one thing, are multilayered, and are usually *about* something – they are a dynamic relation to the world, a form of knowledge, too.[15] The operations of the psyche cannot be *reduced* to their organic dimension: the story of a psychotic patient such as Eric is not wholly encapsulated by his neurobiology, because even the biology is grounded in a story of distress.[16] Yet, given all our complex layers and history, the tools of Kraepelerian psychiatry that are still used today are not adequate for a consideration of the self both as a whole and in relation to others, and as originally defined within the talking therapy established by Bleuler and Freud. Just as psychoanalysis mostly left behind the organic dimension of mind, so psychiatry, its elder sibling, today can sometimes be in a no-man's-land between brain and mind – at once both neurology and therapy, and neither one of them.[17] Eric himself seems stuck in a no-man's-land. He is at once a clinical case and an existential enigma – an instrument of medical methods born of historical and cultural forces he has nothing to do with. His gaze is not just the outcome of his damned chemistry, or of generic or brand names of targeted molecules, or the living demonstration of how data yielded by scientific research on experimental cohorts and population samples tells us something about how the brain works. Eric feels guilty: that dimension – *how* he actually *feels* – matters as much as the pathology that is causing the feeling.

Guilt, again, is a *social* emotion: it involves our relations and actions in the world of others, within a map of moral meaning. Developmental psychology shows that it begins to percolate in humans around the age of two.[18] It is a crucial aspect of our development as morally aware beings, a component of social cohesion, and an element in moral psychology that has its own cultural history and anthropological variations.[19] As a force underlying our relation to others, guilt features widely within psychoanalytical theory as well – for Freud, it is 'the ultimate source of religion and morality', arising out of the Oedipus complex, itself 'one of the most important sources of the sense of guilt by which neurotics are so often tormented'.[20] The Austrian-British analyst Melanie Klein dated the onset of feelings of guilt to even earlier, to infancy, positing that unconscious guilt about feelings of envy and wishes to destroy the

loved object was what enabled the process of psychic reparation.[21] Whatever its sources, however, Eric's feeling of guilt is
an amplification and displacement of an emotion that marks,
and depends on, the boundaries of the self in relation to others.
His guilt questions the foundations of his very existence as a
legitimate being. He can only look up to the heavens, for fear
of looking out at others and of feeling his own abjectness in
his eyes: the grandiosity is a mode of surviving this guilty
abjectness. Eric's slowness may have been a side effect of his
drugs as suggested by the doctors. But his psychotic state is
an extreme expression of what can go wrong in the development of the self – and so also a mirror image of all that must
happen for things to go right.[22]

For it is the social construction of the self – of the self in
relation to others – that is distorted in a psychosis; any psychiatric disorder, for that matter, is a disorder of 'social
interaction'.[23] For Freud, this distortion could be on a
continuum with neurosis, which he understood as an internal
conflict between ego and id, while psychosis was 'a disturbance
in the relationship between the ego and the external world'.[24]
But a view that developed within psychoanalysis after (and
beyond) Freud, notably by Donald Winnicott, asserts, even
more strongly, that our psyche is a function of those around
us.[25] Our social self is commensurate with our biological self:
the self defines itself in relation to the non-self. We can only
become persons by way of others.[26] Recent studies of interoceptive processes, notably by psychologists Aikaterini
Fotopoulou and Manos Tsakiris, reinforce this view. They show
how it is through the infant's relation to its first carers that
we develop as integrated selves.[27] The 'minimal self' – Damasio
calls it the 'protoself' – depends on the sense of our own body,[28]
which in turn begins with those who first hold us as babies:
how we eventually recognize and accept ourselves as autonomous persons and agents depends on how others held and

nurtured us from birth.[29] We are born completely physically dependent, and only develop into independent, self-conscious agents as if from the outside in, our skin eventually the boundary of self only insofar as we are able to recognize as our own the processes going on *inside* our body. This is also why the physical connection to a mother is so strong – as I am experiencing. Our hormones and neurotransmitters, cardiac structure, microbiome, tastes, musculoskeletal structure, joints, pain threshold, levels of sense-perception, and so on, all participate in who we are and how we are in the world of others, with others. Our affective, relational, and narrative self is inseparable from our biological self, from the body that we live in.[30]

Eric's sense of self is fundamentally disturbed.[31] What has gone wrong with him in his psychosis is the opposite of what goes right in the development of ordinarily healthy people, even those with varying degrees of neurosis. The very foundation of his being has become uprooted from the body into which he was born. And so there is a difference in kind, not just in degree, between the ordinary neurotic and the psychotic, and this is what disturbs us. Eric seems akin to one of those 'mad' people that used to be kept in shackles as if they were no longer a person. Ordinary neurotics were never shackled. I don't know what exactly happened to Eric, or what his family history is: the anamnesis gave no information about it (nor, given its summary form, could it have given enough to fathom much in any case). But whatever did happen, and whatever is the matter with him, is biologically manifest: Eric has disturbances in interoceptive predictive signals,[32] and his anorexic appearance is most probably connected to these disturbances, a manifestation of his disordered sense of his embodied self.[33] The emotion of guilt that torments him seems to arise from what he perceives as the inadequacy of this self to meet the world's (imagined) requirements. Sometimes we may punish our embodied selves in order to punish our socially defective selves. We can see here how the biological processes at work are thoroughly enmeshed with how emotional, interactive meaning is made. A grandiose patient such as Eric has a distorted sense of his agency within the world. The grandiosity compensates for his guilt. But it may also be a compensation for the altered (reduced) interoceptive accuracy – the difficulty in detecting accurately his bodily and visceral sensations.[34] Such as he is, Eric can only be disappointed by the world. And there can be no fulfilled life in a world that perpetually disappoints.

There have been attempts at a psychotherapeutic approach to try and unravel the knots that create these disorders, and weaken their hold on the organism. Sicilian psychiatrist Gaetano Benedetti applied psychotherapy to the treatment of psychosis.[35] The practice, which he developed at first in Switzerland and the United States, is not widespread, and it has not been widely studied, but as the rationale for a division between neurology and psychiatry fades, so the range of clinical methods could expand, to help those with extreme, disabling mental distress. It is sobering to realize that, for every psychotic, delusional Eric, there may be many desperate but functioning, neurotic, or angry ones who also believe no justice can be found in this world – unless it be saved by a powerful, redemptive leader, perhaps. For that matter, one deluded individual such as Eric may be far less harmful to society than a large number of angry neurotics. Madness is not beyond the pale: it is on a sliding scale of being.

Eric, however, is also depressed. Severely. Depression is terribly common, regardless of where we come from, who our parents are, or what our story is. While all of these can be factors in predicting a depressive tendency, they do not alone determine its presence or absence.[36] Eric's depression may well be clinically connected to his Parkinson's, as often is the case,[37] but regardless of its cause, one can empathize with his state, because there are very few people who have never felt darkness within at some point or other. In its extreme version, depression is the 'darkness visible' William Styron was one of the first to dare write about with frankness.[38] Anyone can become tangled up in knots so tightly that speech stops. In all its forms, one could say that depression is a condition of being at once conscious and mortal. Melancholy – the word for 'black bile' in Greek – is its noble ancestor.[39] For centuries, the term melancholy covered the whole range of distress, from banal blues to suicidal depression or delusional mania. But episodes of mild depression are very different from the morbid melancholia Eric presents with. Both melancholics and manics come in many guises. A person can undergo a manic-depressive episode once and remain otherwise healthy, or suffer for life from what Kraepelin was the first to name 'maniac-depressive insanity'.[40] It became what we know as bipolar disease, what Kraepelin had seen as a 'relapsing and remitting' condition, in contrast to a chronic one.[41] The two states had been understood already by the first-century Greek physician Aretaeus as twin aspects of one pathological condition, though interpretations of these symptoms fluctuated throughout history.[42] Until modern psychiatry categorized states of mind or being into discrete pathologies, melancholics were often seen as creative, inspired, and capable of artistic transcendence. Melancholy, as the great Robert Burton showed in his *The Anatomy of Melancholy*, first published in 1621, also named obsessives and erudites such as himself, phobics, holy men, monomaniacs, jilted lovers, as well as those who imagined themselves emperors – a variegated ensemble of what today are very disparate neurological disorders, psychiatric conditions, or psychological states, though they are by no means mutually exclusive.[43]

Eric seems to have stepped out of Burton's century. He reminds me of an English religious enthusiast – enthusiasm, from the ancient Greek *entheos*, or possessed by a god, was attributed to those 'inspired' people who heard voices from on high in the form of a direct connection with the specifically Christian Holy Spirit. Seventeenth-century England was rife with such 'enthusiastic' religious sects, broadly branded Puritans, particularly during the Civil War and its aftermath – between the execution of Charles I in 1649 and the ascent to the throne of Charles II eleven years later.[44] Many of them made their way to North America, where these sects thrived and multiplied.[45] By the middle of the century, to be branded an enthusiast in England was not a compliment. The term was associated with pathological hallucinations, and those afflicted were seen as deluded, obsessive, grandiose – dupes driven by the wishful fancy that transcendence was within their personal reach. That wishful fancy still exists, and can take all sorts of forms in which pathology does not figure so explicitly – think of today's sects, for instance, and mainstream evangelicals in the United States. The pathologization of religious enthusiasm began in the eighteenth century, with rationalism and deism: by then, Eric would have been viewed as a prime example of a pathological enthusiast.

In 1691, the Anglican bishop John Moore gave a noted sermon on 'religious melancholy', sufferers of which were debilitated by their obsession with sin. Moore attributed its cause to a disease of the body.[46] Where the religious enthusiast had a vision, the melancholic had an unhealthy fixation. The two conditions were related, and, in an age of secularization of medicine, the sufferers of both were considered to need some sort of medical help. They were afflicted with a disorder of the brain, a form of insanity. Eric's case could have illustrated the 1725 treatise *A Treatise of the Spleen and Vapours: Or Hypochondriacal and Hysterical Affections*, by London physician

Richard Blackmore, who saw the self-condemnation of the religious melancholic as a disease, where, true to the Hippocratic creed, 'all diseases are deviations from the natural rectitude of the constitution.'[47] Hysteria and hypochondria – which Blackmore, true to tradition, gave as the male equivalent of hysteria – could give rise to 'divine prophetic inspirations'. It needed saying, because debates still raged at the time over whether visions, possessions, and inspirations were really caused by the coarse matter of body and brain, or whether demons might not be active, or indeed some visions not legitimate.

Those questions had been put to the test repeatedly over the seventeenth century, famously so in the 1630s by the Ursuline nuns at the French town of Loudun, who claimed they had been possessed by the devil in the form of the good-looking parish priest, who had seduced a few of the nuns. Stories of extorted confessions, of being possessed, of exorcisms riven with sexual innuendo, political manipulation, legal machinations, and of public spectacle eventually led to the priest, Urbain Grandier, being tortured and burned at the stake without the benefit of a secular trial. The claims of witchcraft were later shown to be fabrications. The episode would one day provide fodder for reflection for neuropsychiatrist Gilles de la Tourette (he would give his name to Tourette Syndrome), a pupil of Charcot who was born near Loudun. He annotated the autobiography of the convent's prioress Jeanne des Anges, in which she told her tale of being possessed, and Charcot wrote the preface.[48] But beyond this well-known, much analysed and deconstructed historical episode, the power of popular accounts of witchcraft, devils and possession belies yet again how our self-perceptions are shaped by culturally given beliefs, themselves the products of collective imagination, if not actual collective hallucinations. We create these tales to sustain our emotional needs and justify our beliefs: to fulfill their function, they must be inherently convincing. It is easy to delude ourselves, and even easier if everyone around us shares the same delusion – a psychotic *folie à deux* can be played out in society, and turn into what one may as well term collective hysteria.

Eric, by contrast, is deluded, but he is very much alone – as was Toussaint. He is no sect member. Still, he also reminds me of another type of religious enthusiasm, that of seventeenth-century Jansenism. Jansenists were a sect who based their creed on a posthumous text called *Augustinus*, by Dutch theologian Cornelius Jansen, which tweaked Catholic doctrine so that it resembled Calvinism. Catholics, and Jesuits in particular, deemed it heretical and condemned it.[49] Jansenists actually thought of themselves as Catholics, and would have baulked at being associated with any enthusiasts since their theology was complex and scrupulously thought through. But they diverged from Catholic doctrine in their attitude to the role of human free will in the receipt of divine grace, believing humans had none, given the weight of our original sin. After a 1720 Papal Bull, the Unigenitus, sought to condemn Jansenism, it became more extreme. A Jansenist called François de Pâris, an ascetic of wealthy extraction, opposed the Bull, ending his life at the age of thirty-six by extreme self-flagellation, complete with hairshirt and spiked belt. His tomb became a pilgrimage site at which people began to experience convulsions and miraculous cures. The *Convulsionnaires* were born, a new sect whose members believed in the value of pain and self-flagellation. Some Jansenists defended it, others did not. By the 1740s, the movement had died off.[50] But its popularity shows how attractive complete self-denial can be, and the idea that one's existence can only be lived if one condemns it. It is the opposite of the celebration of life. Yet it is not a declared pathology.

A renowned and admired exponent of Jansenism whose work

has survived these momentary fervours is the great thinker Blaise Pascal, who gave up his scientific passions and practices after meeting a Jansenist doctor who cured his father of a broken hip. His sister had joined the Jansenist convent at Port Royal a few years earlier. His *Pensées* are still read today, for their depth and lucidity.[51] But he was also self-flagellating, and his views can be bleak. Sin was at the centre of his thought, even though he was aware of how shocking the doctrine of original sin was to our reason. It was 'unjust', he wrote, 'to damn eternally an infant incapable of will, for a sin wherein he seems to have so little a share, that it was committed six thousand years before he was in existence', and yet, 'without this mystery, the most incomprehensible of all, we are incomprehensible to ourselves. The knot of our condition takes its twists and turns in this abyss, so that man is more inconceivable without this mystery than this mystery is inconceivable to man.'[52] It is a very particular view of human destiny, another cultural construct that, once it becomes absolute, can profoundly form and determine a worldview, a life, a fate.[53]

Eric feels guilty in a Pascalian sense. He seems a man of God who could have sat at a table with Pascal and discussed his perhaps non-pathological belief in the deep, inherent guilt of humanity. But this belief has merged with an obsessive religious melancholy that Dr Blackmore would have worried about: Eric is indeed psychotic, in modern terms. He is also an oddball. He could be the subway preacher, if he were louder, more assertive, more determined, and less fearful. And he is suffering. That is why he is consulting these doctors. Whatever theological view he adopts to propound his own guilt has nothing to do with the reality of his feelings: it seems that he needs to anchor his *a priori* guilt in a larger, culturally solid context. For he has nothing objective to be guilty about, as far as we know. He hasn't killed anyone, and may not have hurt anyone – although 'hurt' can be relative, and such biographical details are not available. Perhaps his is an extreme form of anxiety, combined with the depression that comes after mania – the terrible down that follows the manic belief that one can achieve anything. He apologizes to us for not having lived up to expectations. We don't know what expectations, exactly. No one expects anything, but he thinks the world did. Maybe that is the problem. I don't know how he ended up at the packing company. Why he didn't take holy orders, become a priest, a preacher, a purveyor of truths to a misguided humanity. But in his mind, his guilt is so large there is no point in trying to get rid of it. It may be more manageable for him as such, paradoxically. Better perhaps to feel on a mission, however failed, than to be prey to pharmacological tricks.

Eric lives, or rather survives, on the edge, standing in what he experiences as the unforgivingly bright spotlight of divinity, at once chosen and damned. And during the session, I asked myself: why is this so interesting, so compelling, to all of us? Are we voyeurs – of others as ourselves, ourselves as others? What are we trying to retrieve here, exactly? The fact is that Eric is deeply recognizable. He reminds me of a Beckett character, and looks like a Giacometti sculpture. Fittingly, Beckett and Giacometti were friends. Both were bony men who loved tobacco and ate little. And my parents were friends with them too – they were Sam and Alberto to them. Neither was literally mad, but each stood on the edge of existence, and on the border of the expressible, struggling with absented gods, Sam sculpting essential words into silence, and Alberto figures out of clay, or plaster, in the process of disappearing. Sam in particular was a central figure in my parents' lives and a central anchor for my father until he died in 1989. (Giacometti died much earlier, in 1966.) Our home life was infused with a constant attendance to intensely subjective perception. And my parents' work was devoted to the exploration of its transcendence, through painting and poetry.

The ability to represent the seen and heard in new form is the work of the imagination. We saw with Vanessa how imagination and memory overlap, the one necessary for the other. What is remarkable with my mother is that the verbally inflected imaginative play endures despite the fading of the mnesic traces without which projection into the future, even the near future, is impossible. The cognitive reserve that seemingly protects her imagination could well be the very 'power' she drew on first to escape the religious enclosure of her family, and then to become a poet. Throughout her life, she turned facts into emotional experiences, and emotional experiences into verse. My father performed the equivalent alchemy, turning the world of things into visual poetry, painting always within the confines of one day, against time, in a state of emergency fitting for the survivor he was – of concentration camps, war, human darkness. As the illness asserted itself, her past life with my father merged at first into her inner dialogues with 'Sam', even as everything gradually faded into a blur, clear lines turning into blobs, prose into verse, not always comprehensible by now – except as slanted, at times insightful, surrealist poetry.

Isn't her unravelling a kind of madness too, besides its cruelly precise neurological etiology? Why is Beckett's bleakness so compelling, and why did Giacometti sculpt those thin disappearing men? How absurd it all is – that it all should end so, and that we should know it. We understand what madness is, for good reason. 'We are all born mad. Some remain so,' says Estragon in *Waiting for Godot*. To look at Eric, I realize, is to look at the other side of life and joy, at what happens when body and self break apart, when the stuff of life cannot sustain itself, when the search for transcendence is misdirected, and falls flat. But both life and transcendence happened, with a

vengeance, in the interstices of Beckett's lines, and within
Giacometti's disappearing, dynamic figures. The texts and the
figures remain beyond death. It is odd to think that I am the
daughter of a man and woman who were their friends, and
who also remain: he within his paintings, she within her words,
which, however lost to her now, are the words she once wrote.
She doesn't know it anymore, but they both achieved transcendence too. Without the gods. My father had seen the abyss,
walking on a ledge every day, living in joy and hope. With a
vengeance. A soft melancholy he shared with Sam nourished
creativity. But from the time of Sam's death, a more brutal
depression hovered too, coming and going, threatening to
undercut the sense that there was any point in going on. 'They
give birth astride of a grave, the light gleams an instant, then
it's night once more,' my father would often quote, from
Waiting for Godot. The light stayed on, always – until night
fell. It is hard to live without the gods. Pointlessness can take
away power.

Eric is not an artist and he does not have access to the
consolation of creativity, but he seeks higher meaning. He also
seeks absolution. At the end of the speech he gave after
returning to the room as the doctors were discussing his case,
an older, retired neurologist seated next to me, a tweed-clad
man with a wise face who sometimes attended the sessions,
spoke up from the back of the room. Taking on the role of
celestial judge, he declared that he, Eric, was absolved of any
guilt. Eric had been able to leave after this: he had received
the absolution he dared not ask for, but which he needed far
more than he wanted any medical help. (The older doctor had
made the declaration instinctively, without thinking about it,
he told us afterwards.) The doctors would prescribe anti-
psychotic medication. But Eric may hold on to his great guilt
for dear life, an unfathomable companion to his slowly creeping
Parkinson's. It may also dissipate. And perhaps he will continue

talking with an unseen dimension that will give his life more meaning, and make it less pointless, than does his job at the packing company. He is a man who, from the depths of despair, and caught within the net of a debilitating illness, needs to look up, even as the world looks away.

Because it is far more convenient, and frankly happier, to look away than to face things head on. Pascal, Jansenists, enthusiasts, and assorted melancholics do not make for light-hearted company. It was a relief to feel the darkness Eric carried into the room dissipate that morning after his departure. The exercise of empathy was spent. The theatrics had been cathartic. Now the Beckettian performance was over. But we all exited the room feeling stunned, as if a rock had been hurled at us, as if we had been made to hear the cries and grief of all suffering humanity – that sometimes seemed echoed in the unstoppable rattling of the blinds outside the room's large windows, when the wind blew. And I realized, later: here I am telling the tales of the disrupted minds of strangers while my mother is losing hers, blessedly laughing all the way.

7

Hold My Hand

I've long since had my tea, my dark, my dawn.
I've done what I thought others asked of me,
though they had not expected all they got;
had not required once
this night my soul
that never will have peace it can afford,
though it wait, it wait.

Anne Atik,

from 'The Next Time', in *Offshore* (1991)

Blessed laughter. My mother's Jewish humour is a part of her. It is preserved now even as her neurotic anxiety, which was such excellent fodder for the humour, is mostly gone. The anxiety was also fodder for her poetry – for lines such as the ones here above from her collection *Offshore*. (A poem in the collection is about her teaching me the Hebrew alphabet, when I was nine. I asked her of late if she remembered it. She said: 'Of course I remember it – I just don't know how to write it!') There was never any psychosis in her story, nor psychiatric distress. Her troubles are unambiguously organic. Neurons turned tombstones – undermining functions, progressively, though their functioning fluctuates.

Dementia is widely studied. This reflects the large number of people afflicted by it. And though all aspects of dementias

are investigated, it is most likely that discoveries on the molecular and genetic levels will have the greatest impact on
medical efficacy. But still, we know little. And however much
science I read, there remains that gap between the precise
accounts and the phenomenon. Between cool explanations
and the lived experience, which includes anything but cool
emotions. The connections between scientific explanation and
lived life are sometimes dizzyingly revelatory, but sometimes
they are non-existent. The predictive processing theory, for
instance, has recently been used to explain the diverse symptoms that people with dementia can exhibit – the memory
disturbance, bradykinesia, apraxia, word loss, misperception
of sounds and words, inappropriate social behaviour, motor
troubles, and more.[1] Yet so far, clinicians can do little with such
an explanation. And families, even less. The brain is too
complex for available neuroscientific explanations to sum up
what happens to the embodied and emotional self in which
some neurons are turning into tombstones.

That my mother's affect remains untouched so far means
that, as is often the case with many patients diagnosed with
Alzheimer's, some integrity of self is preserved for a while,
along with her recognition of those she loves. Positive memory
is resistant: encoded feelings aren't dissolving so readily. We
are able to engage her full emotional attention especially when
we put on music, which was always a central part of her and
my father's lives. Her intensely felt musical memory is intact.
And it seems that musical memory – an aspect of implicit,
unconscious memory, as opposed to explicit, conscious memory
– has specific neural networks, which would explain why it is
often spared dementia's onslaughts even at an advanced stage.[2]
Not long ago she came for a late summer lunch, and I played
a recording of poignant Yiddish songs from the Bund, recap-
tured by a young singer from Vienna. As one song began, my
mother suddenly gasped: 'But I know that!' And she hummed

along, moving her shoulders in tempo, beating her hand on the table, at first moved, then amused. An old world had returned, here and now, in sensorial form, within her body.

An assault on the self's embodied integrity can happen in a myriad of ways. And these ways are often mysterious. I saw many patients, like Vanessa, whose disturbances were hard to locate organically, yet who were suffering enough that they needed to consult the neuropsychiatry clinic. Their disturbances were very different from what is affecting my mother, and pointed to a possible resolution, rather than to the inevitability of terminal decline. But their stories revealed much about brain–body interactions that may enrich our understanding of how dementias are played out throughout the body and the multilayered, somatic memory that constitutes our sense of self and purpose within the world.

Claire was one such patient. When she walked into the hospital room, one could tell that she cared about her appearance. She wore an ochre top tucked into a belted, pleated skirt. We had learned during the anamnesis that she used to set up cultural activities for the elderly, and had been proud of her job. Dozens of local councils had entrusted her with missions that she felt helped give life to these places. It was not particularly glamorous, but it gave her satisfaction. And self-presentation mattered in the role. She had retired a few years before, it was not clear how many exactly – two, three, perhaps four. The last couple of decades had been hard on her. She had been depressed – and in turn agitated. She barely ever saw her children, who found her hostile. She fought with many of her neighbours, who also found her hostile. Mostly, she was afraid. She did not know quite of what, but she knew that she had to protect her right hand from any further aggression.

Twenty years earlier, she had fallen and hurt that hand. Her carpal canal was injured and she was operated on soon after. But she had been in pain ever since. She developed what is

known as algodystrophy, or Complex Regional Pain Syndrome
– CRPS – another way of describing the burning, swelling,
and general hypersensitivity she felt. The pain had even travelled up her arm, to her neck. Her fingers retracted. No
treatment worked. Every single day of her life was marked by
that ongoing, debilitating, infuriatingly distracting pain. Years
passed like this. An EMG detected that a nerve was affected.
Then, just a few years before her visit, there developed strange,
rapid, involuntary movements in her hand and arm, which one
doctor diagnosed as an instance of the fairly rare disease
'myoclonic dystonia', originating in the central nervous system
– myoclonic being the term used to describe involuntary
twitching, and a dystonia being a repetitive motion, due to
muscle contractions. She felt locked into her state.

She was chewing gum when she entered. The injured and
injurious hand was hidden away like a delicate little animal,
wrapped inside a glove, partly hidden inside the crux of her
left arm. She had covered it with a leaflet, possibly an information sheet from a hospital unit. She was rigid, though she
looked youthful for her age, and energetic. She surveyed the
room rapidly with clear, light eyes. 'Imagine if your hand were
cured,' ventured the neurologist after she'd sat down. 'That
would be wonderful,' she replied. 'I could get going again.
That surgeon – because of him I had to stop everything.'
She didn't remember that the surgery had taken place over
two decades before. Her sense of time was askew. When the
neurologist asked her whether her hand was better or worse
now than it had been then, she was unable to answer. But
when he asked her, 'Are you happy or sad?' her immediate,
spontaneous retort was 'happy'. She could not see herself as
one of those sad people. She was still somebody.

Still, she wouldn't uncover her hand. Prompted repeatedly
by the examining doctor, she refused. When he tried, gently,
to take her hand, she became even more rigid, her defenses

up like the quills of a porcupine. She said she rarely dared go out because she feared people would point at her. Her hand was her handicap. And her glove, it seemed, had become a second skin, or armour, though she clearly did not know what the glove might be protecting her from. She once had put her hand in hot water without feeling anything, she told us. She said it seemed to her she had a hole in her hand, instead of a muscle. It retracted itself on its own. If she used it at all, it was always with a rubber glove. She was able to wash dishes in that way, protected by the rubber. She barely had assistance cleaning the house and had turned down her son's offer to help, she said proudly: she managed. And she certainly could not write with her right hand, although she wanted to – and yes, she was right-handed. She had become incapacitated. She was fed up, she said. Disgusted. Exhausted. She also seemed at once aware and not aware of what was going on around her. Asked to name the president, she stumbled. She mixed up words, too. When one of the psychiatrists asked her how life had been twenty years before, she said, 'Life is hard for everyone, I don't know if that is depression, there is no point in remunerating' – she meant 'ruminating'. There was no remuneration in all this, indeed.

Claire left the room after a fairly brief examination, and the discussion began immediately. Her hand, said the psychiatrist, was the repository of all her feelings, the locus of all that had gone wrong, whatever it was. The cause, in her mind, was clear – that surgeon all those years ago. The consequences in her life too. She was convinced the problem was where it seemed to be, in her hand – and now that she had retired, her focus on that hand was all the stronger. But the clarity of this causal explanation seemed to mask some sort of confusion, and to make the problem as intractable as it had become. As another one of the psychiatrists put it, everyone represents their illness to themselves in their own way. To start undoing the process that had led to the gloved hand, one would have to take apart, or deconstruct, the representations she had built of her own inner body. This was not an instance of genetically based 'myoclonic dystonia', said the neurologist.[3] The dystonia was rather 'idiopathic', the term used when the cause of an ailment is mysterious – a disease of its own kind, unexplained. Something had occurred that caused an anomaly in the extrapyramidal motor systems, he continued – the system responsible for involuntary movement.[4] No distraction from her hand helped her. And her basic hostility and terrified defensiveness meant that she had refused to undergo the requisite number of neuropsychological tests. She had difficulty concentrating when stressed – she had admitted as much. The tests that she had done had revealed some degree of disinhibition – and a broadly dysexecutive picture that was probably due to her reluctance to answer the questions.

Claire suffered from a real ailment. But she had no identifiable pathology. It was a disturbance in the functioning of her nervous system, not a neurological disease. In other words, her ailment was *functional*. And that tight, dystonic, overprotected hand had become the locus for all her anxiety, fear and frustration. This was a so-called 'somatoform disorder': it expressed itself via and within the body, and by this point in time, after all these years, it was playing a role in her emotional economy. The dystonia was now a part of her life, but the chronic pain disabled her so much that she would need to undo the hand's literal knots in order to unravel herself. She would need to find out, said one of the psychiatrists, the semiological value of her dystrophy – what this disabling condition signified emotionally and psychically. Hers was a maladaptive reaction to a somatic symptom, an erroneous representation of her own ailment, a set of exaggerated physical sensations that were the upshot of cerebral events, but, as far as one could tell, not of any named disorder.

The case of Claire thus hit against the disciplinary boundaries that the neuropsychiatric unit she was consulting had been created to overcome. But right then and there, it was hard to see how the psychiatrists and neurologists could help. One wanted to shout, 'Take off that glove, Claire! The fear is the problem, don't you see?' Of course nothing of the sort could be said during her examination. It was painful to see that gloved hand, to witness her distress and her stubborn refusal to budge, her hand the very answer to the problem it posed her. Painful disorders such as these, called functional movement disorders, in fact indicate how our emotions are psychosomatic in the etymological sense of the term – at base embodied, felt responses to inner and outer stimuli, and imbued with a valence, that is, a value of good or bad.[5] These ailments are like emotions that have exceeded their remit as indicators of dynamically shifting feeling and turned instead into static tormentors, finding homes in odd corners of the body, the lower back, the gut, the jaw, or indeed, the hand.

An ailment such as Claire's used to be called 'hysteria', then was classified as a 'conversion disorder' before becoming 'functional neurological symptom disorder' in the *DSM 5*, where it is listed under the subheading 'somatic symptoms and related disorders'.[6] Somatic, not psychosomatic. According to the *British Medical Journal*, these disorders, also known as 'somatization disorders', include 'distressing physical symptoms that are not fully explained by other medical, neurologic, or psychiatric disorders.'[7] The changes in classification and naming reflect a change in the mechanisms that are thought to be involved and that need to be understood in order for any diagnosis, treatment or prognosis to be envisaged – even as the precise causes remain hypothetical. The term 'conversion disorder' referred to the transfer from the mental to the physical – a psychosomatic phenomenon par excellence. But that designation of 'conversion' has been replaced in the *ICD-11* by 'Dissociative neurological symptom disorder',[8] as well as modified in the *DSM 5*. During the revision process that led to the preparation of the latter, the American Psychiatric Association issued a list of points to note the changes in terminology and classification. It stated: 'Criteria for conversion disorder (functional neurological symptom disorder) are modified to emphasize the essential importance of the neurological examination, and in recognition that relevant psychological factors may not be demonstrable at the time of diagnosis.'[9] In other words, the psychological aspect has now been excluded in the absence of any evidence that this causes the disturbance.

There are no evident neurological lesions in conversion, either – indeed their absence is a central criterion for diagnosis. But the nervous system is clearly in play. Conversion may involve the emotional centres in the brain's thalamic structures, which evolved to respond to environmental cues and menaces, and are activated when one is in a state of high alert, inducing a response of fight, flight, or freeze.[10] Normally such a state is short-lived, and lasts only as long as the environmental menace is present. But it would seem that in conversion disorder, this automatic, evolutionarily ancient response is prolonged after the triggering trauma. Claire had been stuck on the freeze response ever since her fall and surgery, within a well-known post-traumatic mechanism that would have explained the dystonia, and which persisted long beyond the initial, localized trauma. Such patients are as if stuck on survival mode: brain areas that process salient emotions remain persistently activated, leading to the negative emotions becoming entrenched.[11] In Claire's case, the catalyst would have been the fall and surgery – but this psychological element is only a part of the mechanism; it is not a cause.

Claire's ailment could at first, then, seem psychosomatic, at once *psyche* – mind, or soul – and *soma* – body. These ailments are liminal: at once visible and invisible, graspable and ungrasp-able, pathologies yet not, physical yet not, mental yet not. Psychosomatic ailments are common occurrences. As Michel de Montaigne admitted in one of his *Essays*, 'I am one of those by whom the powerful blows of the imagination are felt most strongly. Everyone is hit by it, but some are bowled over. It cuts a deep impression into me,' and 'When I contemplate an illness I seize upon it and lodge it within myself.'[12] Montaigne goes on to describe instances of what we call today the placebo effect, which is powerful enough that double blind trials of medications must take it into account.[13] Today we also call a physiological reaction to acute stress 'psychosomatic' – for instance, the intestinal disturbance or backache that strikes just before an important event, or the various aches and pains, general malaise and fatigue that tend to accompany depres-sion.[14] It is on a continuum with the physiological feeling states that arise out of emotional processes.[15] At any rate, it is more common and banal than the prolonged functional neurological disorder Claire was suffering from, which was of the kind we met with Vanessa.

But to be diagnosed with a functional neurological disorder according to the criteria listed in the *DSM* 5, the patient, as stated in the *BMJ*,

> must have excessive thoughts, feelings, or behaviors related to the somatic symptoms or associated health concerns as manifested by at least one of the following: dispropor-tionate and persistent thoughts about the seriousness of one's symptoms; persistently high levels of anxiety about health or symptoms; excessive time or energy devoted to these symptoms or health concerns.[16]

There is no attempt here at an explanation for the anxious fixation, or at accounting for it in relation to the functional ailment. Yet conversion disorders are, in fact, a type of psycho-somatic ailment, insofar as a potent psychological component is inherent in their *mechanism*, even if they are not *caused* by overt psychical distress. Neurologists who encounter cases such as Claire's tend to send them to psychiatrists. But the disturbance is not clearly psychiatric either.

And so these cases remain hard to grasp, partaking at once of medicine and of psychology, and belonging to neither, though they do fall within the purview of neuropsychiatry. A large number of distinct ailments, in fact, are categorized as neurologically unexplained: dystonia is a particular one, as is CRPS, both of which combined in Claire's case. Others include fatigue – when it is called Chronic Fatigue Syndrome – movement disorders of various kinds, bowel disorders usually grouped under the umbrella term Irritable Bowel Syndrome, or the broad category of dissociative symptoms such as depersonalization, where experience does not feel like one's own.[17] These symptoms can be debilitating in both their duration and their intensity. They have a disruptive effect on people's lives. They are also fairly common – and often are not taken seriously by physicians. The onset of some of these syndromes may follow viral infections, and at the time of writing, increasing numbers of people who have been infected by Covid-19 are reporting chronic symptoms that may be the expression of systemic inflammation, stress reaction and resulting dysfunction of the sympathetic nervous system, and which may lead to some of the physiological responses these patients report.[18]

Mechanistic medicine is no match for these ailments, which require an organismic, multi-system view. Excepting body-centred therapies, there are few specialists in conversion disorder within mainstream medicine. A noteworthy exception is Germany, where there exists a specialty of psychosomatic medicine independent of psychiatry, which incorporates psychotherapeutic principles.[19] But in other countries, the definition of conversion disorder is hazy, though its etiology is increasingly studied. And treatment possibilities are heterogeneous, consisting in practices that are still considered 'alternative' to mechanistic medicine, insofar as they home in on the mind–body nexus, whose centrality to the disease process is acknowledged by the German medical establishment but not yet elsewhere. For that matter, it is hard to identify which existing disciplines could most optimally treat and best study these ailments. What sorts of experiences are they and how can they be made sense of? Siri Hustvedt explored exactly this question in her *The Shaking Woman or A History of My Nerves*, a book that begins as a quest to explain her own, mysterious episodes of shaking. 'The search for the shaking woman,' she writes, 'is also a search for perspectives that may illuminate who and what she is. My only certainty is that I cannot be satisfied with looking at her through a single window. I have to see her from every angle.'[20]

I tried at first to look at Claire from the angle of neurology and felt that something was missing. Historically, neurology has concerned itself with organically based, structural issues such as dementia. And in a case such as Claire's – one of functional neurological symptom disorder/conversion/ hysteria – there are no visible, causative neurological lesions, just as with Vanessa. The *DSM 5* definition of this disorder seems to have emptied it of all explainable pathological content, unmooring it from its very history.

Arguably, Freud's studies on hysteria are a turning point in that history. For twenty years, let us not forget, he had contributed substantially to the neurology of his day, notably in his work on aphasia.[21] But by the 1890s Freud had moved away from the efforts of the time to found a scientific basis for psychology, believing physiology was not developed enough to explain the mind. In this he was following the route of Nancy-based neurologist Hippolyte Bernheim, the foremost critic of Charcot's notion that hypnosis concerned hysterics in particular (Freud had translated both Bernheim and Charcot into German). Pierre Janet, Charcot's ally, pitted himself against Bernheim.[22] As we saw earlier, Freud eventually came to surmise that hysterical states were somatic manifestations of inner conflicts that could be resolved by bringing them verbally to awareness. In *Studies on Hysteria*, he and Breuer hypothesized that hysterical symptoms emerged when a trauma caused a 'hypnoid state':

> in hysteria groups of ideas originating in hypnoid states are . . . cut off from associative connection with the other ideas, but can be associated among themselves, and thus form the more or less highly organized rudiment of a second consciousness, a condition seconde. If this is so, a chronic hysterical symptom will correspond to the intrusion of this second state into the somatic innervation which is as a rule under the control of normal consciousness. A hysterical attack, on the other hand, is evidence of a higher organization of this second state. When the attack makes its first appearance, it indicates a moment at which this hypnoid consciousness has obtained control of the subject's whole existence, it points, that is, to an acute hysteria; when it occurs on subsequent occasions and contains a memory, it points to a return of that moment.[23]

This theory was the initial basis of Freud's psychoanalysis. He progressively established a semiology of affect, a kind of dictionary by which to read into behavioural, verbal, and physical symptoms the signs of a psychic disturbance, on the assumption that the embodied person somehow 'converted' mental distress into a physically manifest form. This is how hysteria, which Freud understood as a psychopathology and as a symptom of repression, first became known as conversion disorder, with the 'intrusion' he and Breuer wrote of being the phenomenon of conversion. And this is the story that has come to an end with the *DSM 5*, even as the absence of neurological lesions in these cases, coupled as it is with the presence of neurological symptoms, continues to baffle clinicians. Officially, the psychological dimension of functional neurological symptom disorder is no longer a defining aspect of it, despite its emotional component – and as if emotions were not part of an overall psychic economy.

Remember that the very term hysteria comes from the Greek for womb, *hystera*: in Hippocratic medicine, the disorder was attributed to a moving womb, and was thus a specifically female condition, connected to the retention of menstrual blood. In many cases it called for sexual activity to disperse the toxic vapours that unsettled the brain and caused the problem.[24] Hysteria has a long, rich history, perhaps in part because for so long it designated behaviour that was beyond the pale and called for containment – wildness, revolt, revulsion, ecstasy, feminine power and rage, the female body itself, so menacing to male-formed and male-ruled institutions. The border between what is seen as pathological and what is considered socially, psychologically unpalatable has always been unclear: the story of hysteria is a social as much as a medical one.[25] The hysteric in full crisis is strange and unattractive – the Hippocratics described symptoms of suffocation, loss of voice, paralysis, sometimes even loss of consciousness. During the Renaissance, hysteria, like epilepsy or certain versions of melancholy, could be confused with demonic possession, and vice versa – hence the witchcraft trials, and, later, the episode at Loudun.[26]

By the eighteenth century, the phenomenon was no longer an exclusively female malady, since hypochondria entered the scene: hysteria was now explained as originating not in the uterus but in the brain and nerves.[27] Hypochondria, originally the name of the abdominal region, also denotes the syndrome of imagined illnesses such as those described by Montaigne. Earlier even, in the seventeenth century, Charles Lepois, a physician much quoted by Robert Burton and known as Piso, was probably the first to suggest the equivalence between hysteria and hypochondria, in a treatise on the subject published in 1618.[28] Thomas Willis, the physician who coined the term 'neurologie' and whose *Cerebri anatome*, first published in 1664, revolutionized neuroanatomy with its extraordinary illustrations of the brain by the architect Christopher Wren, followed suit.[29] In 1683, the physician Thomas Sydenham published in a letter to a fellow doctor, William Cole, a dissertation on the matter of hysteria, which he viewed as a 'chronic', as opposed to an 'acute' disease. 'It resembles,' he wrote,

almost all the diseases poor mortals are inclinable to, for in whatever part it seats itself, it presently produces symptoms as belong to it, and unless the physician is very skillful, he will be mistaken and will think those symptoms come from some essential distemper of this or that part and not from any hysteric disease.

It could affect any part of the body – masquerading as any other. Hysterics might also be pretending, thought Sydenham.[30] Many patients with conversion symptoms still meet disbelieving doctors today, for that matter.

But the idea of an 'essential distemper' long remained a characteristic of hysteria and hypochondria. Until the mid-seventeenth century, 'vapours' were a popular explanation for the ailments, believed to result either from the fermentation of what was thought of as female semen, or from the animal spirits of humoural theory. Vapours were a momentary derangement, not a pathology due to the melancholic humour, though the same conditions for their deployment could be present in both. They were especially rife in the upper classes who indulged in unhealthy lifestyles: heavy diets, insufficient exercise and sloth weakened the organism and made it susceptible to the phenomenon of vapours. Pierre Hunauld, a French physician to King Louis XIV, wrote a dialogue about these vapours, set between a young *marquise* called Sophie, frequently afflicted with them, and a physician called Asclebiades (like the Greek Asclepiades of Bithynia, the atomist physician).[31] During an episode of the vapours, digestive processes tended to be perturbed, and emotions were as if automatic – not indexed on environmental inputs, though the latter could exacerbate extreme moods, resulting in vehemence, convulsive laughter, and 'melancholic illusions'. The humoural model of psychopathology that had prevailed for 2,500 years still helped to account for these states. The vapourous version was another way of imagining invisible body–mind byways.

Later, in the eighteenth century, influential Scottish physician and neurophysiologist Robert Whytt, for whom animal spirits were non-existent, replaced vapours with nerves as the causative factor of what we call psychopathological disorders: vapours became an 'illness of the nerves', whose anatomy Whytt showed in 1764 did not allow for the movement of any substance as would have had to have been the case if the theory of vapours was true.[32] The term 'neurosis', in fact, initially named an illness of the nerves, was coined soon after by another Scottish physician, William Cullen, in 1769.[33] Use of the term 'vapour' now tended to refer to excessively leisurely lifestyle rather than to biology. But hysteria remained a very particular ailment whose physiology was an unresolved problem. Proposed treatments were those that the scientific culture made available and encompassed Franz Mesmer's cures by magnetism, which, for a while, were all the rage because of their remarkable success rate due to the hypnotic quality of the sessions' set-up, rather to any real magnetic activity.[34] Charcot's sessions of actual hypnosis at La Salpêtrière hospital – which had replaced the earlier use of electricity – seemed to induce the symptoms of hysteria, giving them an outlet and thereby leading to their dissolution. And Freud, as we have seen, would replace hypnotism with the 'talking cure', in which free association allowed for the release of the repressed material that translated as hysteria. (Its occurrences were deeply tied to circumstances – connected to the social, economic, environmental, and physical traumas wrought by the Industrial Revolution.) A Freudian neurosis was now a psychological matter, not an organic one as it remained for Charcot, who understood neurosis in Cullen's sense. But the opposition between psychological and organic, functional and neurological – an opposition which arose when neurological lesions were first identified, such as the amyloid protein plaques observed by Aloïs Alzheimer, Kraepelin's colleague – has outlived its usefulness, and results in Claire's hand remaining stuck in its glove.[35]

The *DSM 5*'s umbrella category of 'somatic symptom disorders' points to the *soma*, the visible symptom in the body. But in leaving out the psyche one leaves out a constitutive aspect of that very somatic disorder – the person's circumstances and story. It is as if one ignored the emotional state of a child who becomes chronically constipated after the separation of its parents – as if stress, which is an intensely physiological phenomenon, were not connected to conditions within the environment. Psychosomatic ailments are extremely common, because we are emotional beings, evolved dynamic systems whose feelings inform us about the world and connect us to it. And because, as William James had first seen, all emotional events are bodily events, feeling states are a product of internal bodily sensation, and emotion is the sensing of these changes.[36] Any negative feeling or emotion, already in somatic form by dint of its being felt, is apt also to translate at times into a pathology. Psychic stress is bodily stress: it involves activity of the sympathetic branch of the autonomic nervous system, or ANS, and may result in bodily tensions that can wreak havoc on the organism, even playing a role in the development of vascular diseases and, it seems, some cancers.[37] The hypo-thalamus releases corticotophrin-releasing factor, which stimulates the pituitary gland to produce adenocorticotopic hormone, which in turn triggers the adrenal glands to secrete cortisol, all of which contributes to the state we call stress. Other hormonal circuits are involved as well – complex endo-crinological processes are constantly at work under the skin.

Nothing that matters in a human life is devoid of some sort of affective valence – the sense that something is good or bad, emotionally positive or negative, or somewhere in between.[38] My mother still experiences valence. The embodied psyche tells itself stories at varying levels of consciousness that always have an emotional tenor, tone and colour, and serve an emotional and relational need. And indeed no thoughtful psychiatrist today would deny that psychological stressors can contribute to the evolution of functional diseases.[39] The exclusion of the embodied, environmentally embedded psyche from the *DSM* looks like a pre-Freudian return to William Cullen's original definition of neurosis as an illness of the 'nerves' – as if the psyche were a structure divorced from any somatic expression, as well as from the world. But our emotional memories are embodied memories, as Vanessa's story showed us, and as did my mother's response to the Yiddish song, or to most music she knows, for that matter.

Claire's story was very different from Vanessa's, but there are overlaps with it: it too had stopped in time, in her case with the surgery. Claire's attachment to her glove was profound – clearly emotional, immediate, and psychically inflected. She was attached to her own need. The disorder was by now part of her inner order, as it so often is. But that is precisely how one can define neurosis in the post-Freudian sense. Her hand was the literal embodiment of a neurosis. The traumatic event of the surgery, or whatever was associated with it in her mind, had interrupted her inner narrative, which was literally wrapped around her hand – both her hand and her inner time were frozen. And without an inner narrative, we are unable to project ourselves within and into time, to bind present to future out of the past.[40] Claire's narrative had been interrupted by one traumatic moment, her life story as if reduced to the story of her hand, the telling of her self to and through others shut down within what is known as a 'defense cascade' – a sequence of 'freezing, fight or flight, tonic immobility, and quiescent immobility'.[41]

Psychosomatic ailments can be ways of telling our inner stories when there are no conscious words for them – when they cannot be conceptualized, or even represented to the self.[42] They are an expression of the tight fit between conscious or unconscious perceptions, and the physiological processes that underlie our responses to these perceptions – that is, interoception. We sense, monitor and adapt ourselves to the situations we find ourselves in, often without our realizing it: these are the homeostatic processes thanks to which we physiologically adjust to the changing environment, and to which interoception corresponds.[43] These processes include autonomic, hormonal, visceral and immunological functions: breathing, blood pressure, cardiac signals – our capacity for interoceptive access tends to be measured via the heartbeat[44] – temperature, digestion and elimination, thirst and hunger, sexual arousal, affective touch, itches, pleasure and pain. And these in turn affect the central nervous system and higher cognitive mechanisms in a feedback, 'top-down/bottom-up' loop. The central, peripheral and autonomic nervous systems act on each other – higher cognition, bodily and emotional states interacting constantly. All together these interoceptive mechanisms contribute to the constitution of our sense of self at any given point, lying at its core, and they constitute what we experience consciously as affect.[45]

This sense of our embodied self feeds into our body-representations, that is, how we represent our body to ourselves – which is essential to movement, as well as being central to emotional processing.[46] These body-representations are constantly updated by information provided by our senses, allowing us to navigate the world. Our body-representation in turn is based on the sense of proprioception, which is functionally and anatomically connected to interoception – as is also the case for exteroception, that is, the sensory perception of the outside world. All these senses can be manipulated, as has been done to great effect in the Rubber Hand Illusion (RHI), a landmark experiment that has been often replicated and much discussed: keeping one's own hand out of sight, one watches a rubber hand being stroked at the same time as one's own is stroked, with the result that one feels that the rubber hand is one's own, an effect dramatically demonstrated when the person doing the experiment hits the rubber hand with a hammer and the subject almost invariably recoils as if the hand belonged to him or her.[47] The RHI has been enormously useful for research into the sense of body ownership and the related sense of agency – the sense we normally take for granted that my leg, say, is mine, or that I am moving my own arm – and shows that 'multisensory integration can update the mental representation of one's body.'[48] So when information comes from the visual sense that differs from that of touch and from proprioceptive predictions, body-representations are updated to accommodate these incongruous inputs – and the result can be an illusory feeling, such as the RHI, or indeed the feeling of pain in a part of the body that is otherwise healthy. And so, in cases of CRPS such as Claire's, what may also go wrong are the processes involved in the mental representation of the body – a problem in the integration of the sensory and somatosensory signals that normally sustain body-representations.[49] Here as with Eric, what goes wrong may well show us what it takes for things to go right.

Other experiments inducing a change in conscious body ownership have also been shown to result in nonconscious changes in the interoceptive, physiological regulation of the self.[50] Body-representations and emotional states are neurologically connected. With Claire, a combination of factors that translate as interoceptive processes – anxiety, depression, morbid fixation, negative affect – may have helped turn her dysfunctional body-representation into a neurologically consolidated state of being. Her brain would have created the exaggerated physical sensation and response to the perceived discomfort – a 'somatosensory amplification', possibly involving 'abnormal interactions among large-scale neural systems mediating visceral-somatic perception, emotional processing/awareness, and cognitive control.'[51] These cerebral involvements are not what one would characterize as a focal, that is, specifically located, neurological pathology – the stuff of neurology. Rather, they are processes that favour the fixation on internal rather than on external events – the heightened, emotionally rich attention to interoceptive bodily sensations, at the expense of external inputs. The phenomenon is also the mark of depression.[52] An abnormal motor response such as Claire's is therefore connected to emotional arousal,[53] and imaging studies seem to confirm the cerebral processes in play.[54] But it is not clear how, conversely, the abnormal motor response evolves within the person's overall psychic economy and life narrative. Nor is it clear how this kind of emotively valenced disturbance differs from ordinary anxiety, hypochondria (in its modern sense), or generally from ordinary neurosis.

A notion we first encountered with Toussaint's hallucinations, that the brain serves the body by predicting its states and correcting the prediction errors, may (if accurate) be operative here as well, as it is in all interoceptive and proprioceptive processes: Claire's brain was no longer adjusting its errors in mapping its neural representation of her hand in relation to her body, no longer updating properly the relation of the hand to her interoceptively sensed self. The incoming sensations from her hand no longer matched what her brain predicted.[55] Her hand, to which she paid such morbidly focused, heightened emotional attention, enacting a self-fulfilling prophecy of sorts so that it continued hurting, was no longer synchronized with her narrative time.[56] One might say that what was once called hysteria can now be construed as one massive prediction error.[57] Depression itself, which Claire experienced as well, could be construed in the same way, arising when 'the brain becomes pathologically insensitive to prediction error signals and, consequently, less effective in terms of (metabolic) energy regulation.'[58] Uncorrected erroneous predictions impede the organism's existence within time. Memory repeats itself, imagination is disabled, and the future is as if closed off, and with it relationships. There is only a continuous, static, constantly distorted present in which the error perpetuates itself.[59] The body becomes the mind's prison, and the self is isolated, turned in on itself, no longer relevant within the world.

This phenomenon involves a mechanism also found in schizophrenic patients, in whom there is an inability to compare predictions with sensory feedback associated with any motor command, resulting in their disturbed sense of self-awareness.[60] In a healthy brain, there is a match between the cerebrally shaped expectation of sensations experienced during an action one performs, and the actual sensations experienced during that action. The expectation is known as an 'efference copy',[61] and usually matches the sensory input if one is the agent triggering the sensory stimulus.[62] What conversion patients experience as a failure of self-agency over whatever part of the body is affected – for instance, their inability to lift their arm as they wish to – may be a mismatch between the efference copy and the actual input. (This also explains why we can't tickle ourselves: the brain can predict the effects of one's own hand attempting to tickle, but not those of another. Schizophrenic patients may thus be able to engage in self-tickling when they do not experience their actions as their own.[63]) This deficiency in the sense of agency may be the element that unifies these variegated disorders, connected to the faulty emotional processing, insofar as it accounts for the loss of ability for motor action to follow upon the will to act.[64] And as Damasio had first recounted, we cannot act properly without our emotions informing us accurately about the world and our position in it.[65]

All these theories are only models, of course – interpretations of given sets of data, analysed within specific constraints, in constant development, and only as good as their explanatory power and usefulness. But treatments can be devised on the basis of what we know about interoception: they involve various mindfulness techniques that help patients develop deeper awareness of their interoceptive and proprioceptive sensations.[66] There are also psychotherapeutic practices that could make sense of Claire's plight, according to their own assumptions, with their own semiology. Psychophysical practices are the first-line treatments for conversion disorder, since they provide a way consciously to act upon interoception – as does yoga. Sound-feedback therapy[67] and affective touch[68] have recently been shown to help patients afflicted with CRPS by helping to change interoceptive input. These, and cognitive therapies too, may access the embodied unconscious, or the unconscious body, as well as the paradox and emotionally charged meaning of no longer being the agent of one's body. But they rarely encounter neurology other than via limited efforts to develop a dialogue between neuroscience and psychoanalysis, as with the hybrid field of 'neuropsychoanalysis', launched in the early 2000s by neuropsychologist and psychoanalyst Mark Solms.[69] The diagnosis of conversion disorder otherwise tends to remain stuck in between the tectonic plates that are the various disciplines looking at the mind–brain.

And so, despite the availability today of sophisticated and convincing neuropsychological explanations for what may have happened to Claire, she was another patient stuck in between disciplines and clinical departments, just as her hand was stuck within her glove – and she, within her inner time. She was also stuck within nomenclature: labelling a disorder does not necessarily explain a state of illness, or even define it as an illness. Conversely, a pathological state of mind can be hard to name, especially if its appearance is progressive, as in the case of dementia. A medical name is not a natural kind, meaning that it does not point to the essence inherent in an illness – just as a person who is unwell, like a conversion patient such as Claire, doesn't necessarily have a recognizable disease.[70] At any rate, her resistance to taking off the glove was all the stronger that its symbolic ability to protect her was fragile. Her attachment to it, similar to that of a child to its comfort blanket, was the fulcrum of what a therapist would try to work on to help put an end to her distress, which she alone was causing. She, but not she, exactly: that was the problem. She needed to recuperate her agency, if that was ever to be possible – to recover her hand as her own and thereby get a literal and metaphorical grip on her life. But first, she would have to take off that glove. The question she left us with was if, how, and when she would be able to do so.

She certainly needed help in order to free herself from her self-made prison, where time had stopped and she was confined within an exiguous cell. Such help would have to come from the sort of collaboration between disciplines, departments, and colleagues that was on display at the neuropsychiatry unit. But even so, functional disorders and localized neurological ones such as the dementia afflicting my mother do differ – even if there can be some overlap – in symptoms and in discrete organic processes or dysfunctions. In this regard, the respective remits of the two disciplines does legitimate their separate existence, for the purpose of practical care at least, which explains why it is so difficult for a patient such as Claire to find her place in the medical world. There may not exist psychiatric disorders without an organic component, even an undetected one, but psychiatry is not necessarily relevant to all neurological ailments.

Pointedly, it is not relevant in my mother's case. Her state is due to focal lesions of the brain, and the fluctuations in her cognition and mnemonic ability point to the brain's plasticity, its capacity to re-create lost connections – though at any given time there are more connections lost than there are re-created. Whatever its origin, neurodegeneration is causing the changes in her mental landscape. She is slowly absenting herself within a growing, tentacular amnesia. And she cannot know this. Unlike Claire, she cannot compare herself with all she was before, because all she was before is disappearing. Her temporality is mixed up and reconfigured constantly, while I watch the ravage to her brain cells within the unforgivably linear, unforgiving temporality of normal cognition. At least music recreates bits of world, a last bastion of shareable meaning and temporal order – just as musicality is perhaps also the infant's first mode of access to the world of sounds.

Back to the beginning, then. For now some cogent verbal fragments survive the onslaught, especially expressions of clearly felt affection. The neurologists cannot do any more for her than they can for Claire. We know a lot, and we know very little. We know that in both cases, interoceptive signals are misdirected. In both cases, self-updating becomes jammed, and the body's time becomes disconnected from the world's time. Time is, indeed, of the essence: we construct it, just as we construct our sense of self, our perceptions, and our sense of a continuum. But sometimes, what we construct can come undone, and be unravelled.

8

Impostors

And now in age I bud again,
After so many deaths I live and write;
I once more smell the dew and rain,
And relish versing. Oh, my only light,
It cannot be
That I am he
On whom thy tempests fell all night.

George Herbert, from 'The Flower',
in *The Temple* (1633)

My mother is mostly living within a pure present. It is as if she had achieved the goal of meditation: to counter the constant buzz of the embodied mind, to neutralize drives and desires, to free the self from the ego's despotic rule, find serenity in the here and now, and arrive at pure being, pure consciousness. She is at that place where time stops, where thoughts about the temporal and spatial elsewhere are left to be, where thought itself is stilled. Anxiety is gone. Guilt is not even a distant memory, since there are so few memories. She always had lashings of the legendary Jewish guilt, of the earthy, psychological sort relating to other people – and a very different breed from Eric's metaphysical, Christian one, which involved how he saw himself before God. She would often say that if she didn't feel guilty, 'something must be wrong'. Now she mostly feels gratitude,

benevolence and appreciation. Everything and everyone is beautiful, and 'just as it should be'. Life is simplified, like a return to
childhood – which includes occasional caprices very like those
that children can have, storms within an absolute present. It is
the gradual unwinding of everything that is gradually wound up,
of all the accumulated stuff that sums up a grown-up, lived,
examined life full of thoughts, passions, representations, relations
and interactions. The stuff that I still hold on to, the stuff that
informs my wish to understand the mind, her mind, my mind,
and to write these very pages – all that stuff has come away, but
within this state, she feels alive and happy to be alive. Even as
the unwinding continues, and despite the interruption in verbally
mediated discourse, her sense of what it means to be alive is
preserved. And so in some way, this condition is a blessing – for
her, not for us of course, since we have to accept the loss of
shared memories, and of a shared world.

There need not be dementia for the self's integrity to be
jeopardized, and for anasognosia to hold confusion in place. We
are all multilayered, made of our projections into the past and
the future, and it is hard for many of us to achieve what the
dementia is allowing my mother to experience – that is, to live
in the present. Our metacognitive, imaginative, and creative
capacities are, precisely, the problem. Hence the popularity of
meditation and related practices, particularly in our modern, fast
world. Disturbances to the self's integrity can reveal its fragility.
These take many subtle, and not so subtle forms, from the
momentary sense of alienation to a chronic condition, such as
the dissociation that Janet had described – 'an altered form of
consciousness manifested in disrupted integration of psychological
functions'.[1] When a disintegration of this sort happens in an
otherwise healthy person, it may be a way of escaping a traumatic
past or a terrifying present that may recall that past or trigger
anxiety. Experiences of derealization are common – the upsetting
sense that the world is not quite real, our experience muffled,

indeed that the present is as if at a distance, on the other side of a window pane. These are connected to the rarer, and no less disturbing experience of depersonalization – the feeling of being detached from one's own body, self, and experience. Both states can be connected to heightened anxiety, and usually resolve, though there are cases of chronic depersonalization.[2] Anxiety itself can be a chronic disorder, though not necessarily a pathology – in fact it is somewhere on that murky border between normal and pathological, to echo the title of the classic work by historian and philosopher of science Georges Canguilhem, who defined their relationship one to the other: 'There is no life without norms of life, and the morbid state is always a certain way of living.'[3]

I saw quite a few patients come into the room who were in the midst of a quiet personal crisis, but not in any obviously morbid state. Thomas, for that matter, seemed perfectly normal. He was young, about the age of Vanessa – barely thirty-five – and married to Jeanne, who accompanied him to his consultation the day I saw him. Long-haired and bespectacled, she had a light-hearted mien. He was a little chubby, and wore a stylish beard. We learned that he had an eight-year-old son with a previous wife who used to beat him up, and he had successfully fought to be allowed joint custody. But now Thomas was struggling to care properly for him, as well as for the little girl, now a toddler, he had with Jeanne. According to her, he had himself regressed to babyhood – she had even seen him sucking his thumb on occasion. For a year he had been seeing a psychologist who then retired. And Thomas was even more of a mess now. A lot, in fact, was wrong with him.

Things had never been simple for him and he was used to suffering fits and crises, we learned from the anamnesis. He had become epileptic in late adolescence. A few tonic-clonic seizures – the type of epileptic fit also known as 'Grand Mal', which involves all the muscles in the body, with complete absences, a collapse out of consciousness into nothingness, dangerous falls. Oddly enough, though, the EEGs taken when the fits started had never been abnormal. And since his early twenties, the epilepsy had been under control.

Epilepsy was not the reason for his presence here, in any case. He had memory problems: he had forgotten everything about his wedding to Jeanne. Sometimes he didn't recognize his own family. Often he failed to understand long sentences, and felt unable to read. He tended not to respond to questions, such as when the neurologist asked him, upon his arrival in the room, how he saw things and why he was at the hospital. All he could do was blurt out, in a low voice, that he didn't much like it here. He seemed to have no understanding of what had led him to this place. Barely audible, he managed to say that he had no memories. When he looked at photographs, he said they meant nothing to him. He had no idea whether he had always been this way. He was vague and lived in a haze. He mentioned a needle that 'they pricked' into his back (this had been a lumbar puncture) and heat on his forehead (a fever), as if immediate physical sensation had taken the place of considered experience, as if he were an infant who was not able to read the world and its impacts beyond pure sensation, and could only recognize and respond to basic feelings of pain or pleasure. He hadn't slept well the night before, that much he knew. But he had no idea how long he had been in hospital, or what day it was. The neurologist pressed him: 'Has it been a month, or six months, or maybe a week? If I said that you'd been here six months, what would you say?' 'If you say so,' responded Thomas. 'Well, only one can be true: you've been here either a week, or a few months.' 'I said goodbye to my children,' said the confused patient. 'Yes, I am sure you did – but so, how long ago was that?' 'Not too long.' 'Do your memories fade in your daily life?' 'I can't remember what I did yesterday.' His few sentences tended to begin with 'My wife said that . . .'

It had all begun the year before, on a cold December day, the anamnesis had revealed. Thomas had experienced a bout of high fever along with a headache, muscle pains, and general confusion. Since then everything was jumbled. By now he had stopped driving, and after a knee accident, he also had to stop playing basketball, which was his great passion. He had a pain in his neck, and the right arm and right leg were not working properly. Once, not so long ago, during a street concert in a nearby town, his right leg had become paralysed for about half an hour. He was taken to the ER, where his confusion reached an apex: he thought the year was 2008, though he did remember he had two children. When he woke up the next morning, he complained of cramps, and spoke exceedingly slowly. Soon he was able to walk again, however. But there had also been a problem with his right arm for a few weeks before the leg episode – he would occasionally lose his grip on whatever he was holding. Now he preferred to carry his daughter on the left side – or not at all. He also had nasty headaches, and he tired far too easily. It was all so bad that he had given up his job as a stationery shop manager.

There was something infuriating about the vagueness of this man, whose behaviour clashed with his youth and apparent health. Jeanne said, quite matter of factly and calmly, that he usually got up late, after she'd taken their daughter to nursery and, from there, gone off to work. His mother would come over to help with the toddler. But then we learned from him that he was an excellent housekeeper – in fact he cleaned the house obsessively. An aquarium stood in the living room and he was able to care for that too, feeding the fish every evening. That was puzzling too. How did he remember to clean it on time, as he claimed he did, and how could he be so methodical about the house, when he forgot everything else? Then Thomas mumbled something even more surprising, given his sorry condition: he liked to cook. He used recipes from a well-known

French cookery website. And he made quiches and savoury pies – which required a degree of skill and the ability to take account of quantities and timings. Yet when the neurologist asked him, 'How do you make an omelette?' Thomas couldn't answer. He could successfully follow the directions for a complex recipe but he had a hard time working out what it took to make a simple omelette – and here, in the room with the doctors, he could barely read aloud a recipe for beef stew on the cookery website. When the doctor asked him to count, Thomas was lost. He couldn't recall his date of birth, a loss of implicit memory that is very rare – though he did remember his bank card pin number. He could write the word for music, but could not pronounce it. He even invented some words. When asked to recite the alphabet, he failed to understand the question. Nor did he know any longer whether he was right- or left-handed. But when asked to write on the whiteboard, he did so with both hands, and at one point he even wrote upside-down.

Everything was askew – yet there was no evidence of any distinctive illness, observed the doctors after he departed. Thomas's 'patienthood' seemed fabricated, said one, a collage of bizarre neurological symptoms that had no causes and no name, where language, memory, arithmetic, and the ability to adapt socially were all affected. It was a blurred semiology. There was no neurological damage to his speech – no aphasia, and certainly no degeneration. By the end of the examination, in fact, Thomas was speaking better than he had done at the start. His faulty number sense corresponded to no known, labelled neurological ailment, either. His errors were not symptomatic of anything but what seemed a studied incapacity: they required a degree of effort and cognitive control. His omissions were systematic, however messy. Were Thomas presenting with a breakdown in the executive function, he would have been disinhibited to some degree, and automatic functions would have come to the fore. But that wasn't the case. There was a kind of method to the madness. He seemed like a grown-up baby, a man wanting to shed the heavy weight of adulthood and return to a state of infancy. As if he were, in effect, mimicking the infantilizing effects of some sort of dementia. But Thomas was not demented. And it was the absence of a proper, named neurological disorder that, to the neurologists, pointed to a clear, however mysterious presence: Ganser Syndrome.

I had never heard of Ganser Syndrome, and wasn't even sure of its spelling when I heard the verdict pronounced resoundingly by all the clinicians present, neurologists and psychiatrists.[4] Ganser is exceedingly rare. And this made Thomas's case all the more fascinating. Most puzzling to me, initially, seemed the fact that what was wrong with him was that nothing specific was wrong with him. The salient characteristic for this admittedly vague disorder was the approximate nature of Thomas's responses: vague, not entirely wrong but not quite right either. He understood questions and grasped concepts, but was unwilling or unable – or both – to stick to ordered, coherent responses. The impression one was left with was that of a child playing a silly and irritating game with an instructor or parent, seemingly just for the fun of it.

The German psychiatrist after whom this disorder was named, Sigbert Ganser, delivered a lecture in 1897, published in Berlin the following year, in which he described a consultation that was not very different from that which I had witnessed with Thomas: the patient's responses to simple questions of arithmetic, chronology, or animal description, were mostly wrong – but not misguided. The lecture was only translated into English in 1965, though the syndrome was reported in French in 1937, in the journal *L'Encéphale*, by the German-born psychiatrist and medical historian Walther Riese, under the title 'L'Etat crépusculaire hystérique (Ganser)'.[5]

Ganser is a type of dissociative disorder, a rare subtype of the more common kind of occurrences exemplified by the conversion à la Janet we saw with regard to Claire and Vanessa. Its central characteristic is the 'symptom of approximate answers': a twisted mis-answering, an approximate imitation of paraphasia that comes across as a combination of effort and laxity, volition and unwillingness, and which Ganser had described as *Vorbeireden* – which means to speak at cross-purposes. It has also been called a 'conversive pseudo-dementia'.[6] The disorder features in some aspects of surrealism – André Breton referred explicitly to 'l'état crépusculaire', understanding it as an instance of simulation.[7] The syndrome first made it into the *DSM*'s third edition, which was published in 1980, but it is not included in the current *DSM 5*, published thirty-three years later.[8] The question arises whether one can pin down Ganser Syndrome with enough specificity for it to constitute an illness one can investigate – especially as it seems to originate in a person's need to create an illness, a deformity, the inner monster born of a real imbalance in equilibrium and homeostatic regulation. At once active and passive, someone such as Thomas is a liminal patient. He does not actually wish to be ill as is the case with a patient with Munchausen Syndrome – an equally rare psychiatric condition in which the desire to be ill or injured prevails.[9] And he is not a malingerer who studiously invents symptoms in order to receive medical attention.[10] But insofar as his symptoms are approximate mimicries of neurological deficits or psychiatric conditions like schizophrenia, they are not symptoms of anything but the psyche at work upon its embodied nature.

The patients Ganser saw and reported on were prisoners. This in itself, and the associated need to defend oneself against a hostile environment, may have provided fertile ground for the development of their symptoms, which included hallucinations and what he called a 'clouding of consciousness'.[11] Riese also saw it as a defensive state that tended to occur when one feared punishment of some sort. A psychiatrist in the hospital room recounted, after Thomas had left, the story of a patient who mimicked Huntington's Chorea – a usually inherited neurodegenerative disease – so completely that he ended up in diapers. Referred to therapy, he was eventually able to recall his history of sexual abuse, and, after a bout of depression, exited what, in effect, had been a conversion disorder. But as Ganser noted and Riese echoed, besides emotional trauma there can be a host of triggers for such an occurrence – which, by all accounts, does not last, and is forgotten after it is over, blanked out as in the dissociative amnesia Vanessa had experienced. These triggers can be dementias, traumatic brain injuries, meningiomas, stroke, an asthma attack, alcoholism, or indeed epilepsy. Some sort of shock, at any rate, does usually precede the onset of this conversive episode. And perhaps not surprisingly, a neurological event usually accompanies it: we know from EEGs that it can present with cerebral hypo-metabolism – a decrease in cerebral activity, as evinced by a decrease in a brain area's consumption of glucose.[12] In the case of Thomas, but also in other cases that have been noted, the hypometabolism was seen in the posterior parietal cortex, reflecting the associated deficits in attention to the here and now, the strange sense of vagueness, the absent presence, or present absence, of the Ganser patient.[13] Riese described the condition as a 'general perturbation' that manifested in para-phasias, aphasia, visual agnosia, and the like, none of which pointed to any organic or psychogenic origin. It also came with a 'complex intellectual behaviour' where objects acquired a symbolic value and thought itself became symbolic and detached from concrete reality. It was ultimately an unstable, labile *'dissociation of consciousness'* (his italics) that came and went, and that caused suffering, producing behaviour that, as he put it, was 'not even infantile'.[14]

Once this diagnosis was arrived at, it became possible to re-interpret Thomas's brief, early history of epilepsy as an acute dissociative fit that augured his current dissociated state, rather than as a real case of Grand Mal. And it occurred to me how peculiar this current dissociation was, how it was that Thomas had partially disappeared, ceased to inhabit the self which he had been. No one body area was the site of dissociation, as in the case of Claire and her hand. Instead, it was the very relation between self and world that had gone askew, as if neutralized by a generalized vagueness that had an effect on the simplest cognitive operations. His was the story of a crisis, an interruption of ordinary life, a careful albeit partially unwilled deconstruction of all that it takes to exist as an autonomous agent. It was odd to watch someone performing without realizing that he was doing so. His mistakes were not signs of incapacity, but signals of a capacity to construct a syndrome. They revealed that Thomas's problem was the very fact of the performance of that problem – the manifestation and enactment of a clouded mind, rather than of a specific neural disturbance. There may have existed a real memory deficit over which, indeed, he had no control, and for which cerebral modifications might be found, but there was also an element of volition within the loss of control. Thomas had unwittingly fabricated the dissociation between voluntary control and automatic behaviour – hence the displayed inability to count properly, for instance. It seemed a way to transcend a fear of insignificance by becoming significant – Thomas had a modest life and made few demands of it or himself – adopting illnesses that seemed to be about the self, but instead voided the self of any meaningfulness, utility and connectedness. He effectively brought himself back to a baseline – that of helpless, 'not even' infant or helpless pseudo-patient, all the more helpless because the patient was not suffering from any ailment other than having to be himself.

Yet Thomas wanted to be a proper father again. He wanted his simple life back, his unambitious work, his future. During his examination, he did recall a before that he wanted to return to. He even wanted to understand what was going on. 'I want my neurons back,' he said. He did not enjoy his slowness. He couldn't bear the headaches and the tiredness. Eventually, though, like all Ganser patients he would exit his 'crepuscular' state and emerge back into his adult, functional self, having forgotten all about the pathological state his mind had sculpted into his whole being. It is significant that the condition comes wrapped inside an eventual amnesia about its occurrence – as if it were a phantom state whose very condition is an absence, the forgetting of which at once enables and signals its resolution.

Not all ill-being is illness, but all ill-being is a deformity of sorts that can feel like an inner monster. It is a rupture in harmony, a malfunctioning of those mechanisms we take for granted most of the time, that enable us to live our daily lives in synchrony with the outer world. As a result, the ill or ailing self differs, both physiologically and experientially, from the healthy self. It is in this sense that my mother's dementia is an illness, however 'well' she is otherwise. There are quite a few stories involving people who are tumbling due to weakened limbs, faulty proprioception and messed-up interoceptive signals, the coherence of a usually self-evident self suddenly in question, decomposed into unrecognizable parts. In such stories, emotions become divorced from corresponding actions, social communication breaks down to some extent. Those who undergo these experiences, like Thomas, can come across as impostors, functional but incoherent, their identities unfixed, the gravitational force that centres most of us most of the time turned into a black hole into which wholeness disappears. The process can yield a terrible spectacle of uncanniness.

I saw an extreme case of uncanniness in action, once, in the hospital room. It was an early spring day, chilly but bright, the sky blue above the white modern buildings at the back of the hospital. The patient we were to see was in his mid-forties. We learned from the anamnesis that he was constantly in conflict with another person – within himself. In other words, the other person was an 'alter', and this was a case of 'multiple personality'. It has been known since the fourth edition of the *DSM* as Dissociative Identity Disorder, or DID, though the *ICD* preserves both appellations.[15] The phenomenon is notoriously fascinating, all the more so because its very legitimacy as a disorder is unclear, and its status complex.[16] It has been much discussed since Janet himself, who in 1907 'spoke of abnormal mental integration of the different contents resulting in a lack of integration among two more "*systems of ideas and functions that constitute personality*".'[17] DID is rare, possibly as rare as Ganser – and so the psychiatrists in the unit had deemed this man merited attention, even though, in all probability, the neurologists could not do much for him.[18]

Louis was tall, mild-mannered, quick-witted and, unlike Thomas, very present. He wore a black sports jacket and black shirt, and fashionable wire-rimmed glasses. Nothing in his attractive appearance betrayed his state, or his story. We learned through the anamnesis that he was the result of an accidental pregnancy that occurred when his Brazilian mother was seventeen. There was no father in his life, and little family, apart from a much younger brother he barely saw. He had had occasional moments of absence, and once had an out-of-body experience. As a result, he had been on anti-epileptic medication for a while – no longer, though, as his EEG showed no sign of epilepsy. His MRI was normal as well. But there had been a tragedy some six years before: his wife of eight years, Tania, had died of a brutal cancer, aged barely thirty-five. Shortly after, Louis had tried to kill himself. By now he had stopped working as a computer programmer. He had also stopped playing tennis professionally, following a bad fall that had put him in a coma for a few hours. Latterly he had developed chronic pain in his left knee. As a result he could no longer drive. There was more: both his legs tended to move jerkily at times, as if of their own volition. Louis attributed independent will and emotions to them. It was a case of 'diagonistic apraxia',[19] where the brain's right hemisphere issued a command to the limb that differed from what the normal movement on the left would do – and vice versa. And his right arm sometimes contracted without his will. Only by following a certain, ritualized finger order, could he unlock it, as he showed us; he would unfold one finger at a time, concentrating on each one as he did so.

By the time of this visit, however, things were almost looking up for Louis. He was no longer desperate. He had a new girlfriend, Caroline, and was trying to develop a new web business. But Tania was on his mind, all the time. He replayed her death constantly. He felt he couldn't move on, he told us – and he was very self-aware as he recounted his difficulties. As he put it himself, there was a pessimistic Louis who felt stuck, and an optimistic Louis who wanted to live and enjoy his present life with Caroline, his new vocation, think ahead to having a child, indeed think ahead to everything – but he felt perpetually pulled back by the other Louis. At first sight this did not seem particularly odd: all of us are made of many parts. There are multiple aspects to the self, many self-contradictions within a psyche.[20] But Louis alternated between the two states as if they were two separate individuals, the one actually addressing the other in the second person, for a few minutes at a time. He had become unable to integrate both into one, to tolerate his inner multiples. The conflicted inner conversation was disturbing enough that it interfered with his sleep. His narrative self was divided, incoherent – as if his episodic memory had yielded two very different stories. He was supremely dissociated. And Louis knew that. His optimistic side had grown over the past few years, he told us, enabling him to start perceiving his self-created condition rather than merely enacting it and enduring the presence of the 'alter' passively. He was now self-aware enough to describe how an 'explosion' within himself had happened after Tania died. He was motivated in his life, but stuck. 'Someone else is in the way, another person who doesn't want to move forward.' He, the optimistic Louis, described his experience calmly and lucidly: 'If I let the other person talk, it's negative, not the same person. We are a conflict. At one point he'll take over and I'll stop everything.'

And then, all of a sudden, in the midst of his testimonial, that other Louis emerged before our eyes. It was stunning. The shift happened over a fraction of a second. His voice changed, and he was now the person who wished to continue mourning:

'I lived with Tania eight years, we were good together, why doesn't he understand that I'm in pain, that he's moving forward too fast, why does he want to make a future with someone else, I need time, not a magic wand!'

'We have this project, and he doesn't want to move forward, Caroline is a new dream, why are you stopping us?'

'Well because you don't listen to me.'

The pessimistic Louis was in the room for about ten minutes. Then he returned to his initial self. He told the neurologist he could feel when 'he' arrived, in the form of 'a sensation of tears'. There was nothing he could do about it. It just happened. 'We had another altercation during the night.' The pessimism of that other Louis was menacingly destructive of all he wanted from life. Whenever 'he' emerged, he would point to Caroline, telling him he was standing in their way. He managed to ignore the fact that 'he' was also him. That there was no other Louis

– except that there was. The one created the other, and vice versa.

The neurologist enquired about his limbs, which seemed quite normal just then. Louis described how in fact his legs moved when he was lying down – one foot would move up, another down. And at a certain angle, he had no control over his right hand – he had forcibly to straighten it. 'I'm still not in control of it. And the left leg didn't follow when I got up to walk earlier, I almost fell over.' Significantly, it had never occurred to him that the independent-seeming limbs and the divided personhood could be connected – he had not noticed that he spoke of each in the third person, and addressed them each in the second person. Yet this was clearly the key to his predicament. During the analysis that followed his departure from the room, everyone agreed that the dissociation of limbs and self were part of the same phenomenon.[21] Each had become a separate entity that he had objectified and to which he spoke as if they were not part of himself, and he could only unlock his fingers by commanding them to do so via a ritual external to the self whose fingers these were. He had the dissociative method off pat, though he seemed increasingly able to contain the sad, mourning Louis. It was as if he reified emotions into personas, creating another Louis and independent limbs, his self de-centred from his body, his very coherence as an embodied unity in question. He had relegated pain to another self, cutting himself off from his own past and with it parts of his own body. He had found a balance in which he was – knowingly – trapped, thanks to which he could remain in denial over his inability to mourn, and if he sought clinical consultation and accepted all medical advice, it was precisely because it had no impact, as the psychiatrist noted. He was so well defended, nothing would change without a precisely directed therapy that would cut through the security barrier he had created around his suffering self.

In order to free himself, the psychiatrist thought Louis would first have to become aware that the conflict he had objectified and externalized as if he were a couple of actors in a play was in fact internal to himself. And to help him achieve such awareness, the clinician could begin by taking Louis's internalized drama seriously, sitting the other Louis down in a chair when he was in a depressed mode, and treating him. He would ask him to integrate the negative thoughts in order to reconcile both persons, or sides, or at least minimize his recourse to the dissociative method. It seemed that Louis had always had a tendency, even as a child, to split off his conflicting emotions by play-acting, but, until the death of Tania, he had functioned well enough, and had always felt unified. DID can indeed occur after trauma, and can follow some sort of abuse or neglect in childhood. An explanation for this is that without a secure attachment between child and carers, without the sense that he or she can be safely contained, the child becomes unable to process and regulate emotions. This is the basis of the influential attachment theory of British psychoanalyst, psychiatrist and psychologist John Bowlby.[22] According to this theory, dissociation is a performance of sorts, a means of obtaining some sort of affective fulfilment, with the development of different personas as a defense against the inability to cope with certain emotional states or painful situations or memories.[23] Louis's vulnerability as a child may have laid the foundation for dissociation to occur after the major trauma he had undergone as an adult. We did not know this – his early history was full of gaps and not clearly told in the anamnesis – but in any event, he would have to learn how to reassure himself in order to achieve some normality, and move on as he wished to do.

Trauma is sadly common, not only in times of war but also, more quietly, in times of peace, because violence and neglect can occur anywhere, any time. Its impact on the relationship between body and mind continues to be studied, and has been enriched by growing research on emotions, interoception, and body-ownership. According to the psychiatrist Bessel van der Kolk, traumatic events that may trigger the kind of dissociation that occurs in DID are those in which one has been unable to react, for instance, to an assault, and immobilized in terror. The victim loses the sense of safety normally enjoyed when social relations are reciprocal and mutually attuned. Either an emotional numbness or a hypervigilance sets in, hindering the enjoyment of life and the possibility of intimacy. Memories can be replayed and reinforced, even nonconsciously.[24] The whole organism is as if set in a stress response perpetually present and conditioned by the traumatic event.[25] Broadly put, DID may occur where a protection of the self turns into a multiplication of mutually exclusive, often variegated and numerous 'alters', each of them harbouring its own set of memories, and corresponding to emotions that must be set apart and reified in order to be contained and controlled.

Louis had split himself into two identities. And his two sides communicated with each other, unlike some more extreme occurences in which the various 'alters' or personalities are compartmentalized. He was also aware of the fact that this annoying other Louis emerged out of his need at once to mourn and to put an end to mourning. The question remained why he had reacted in this specific, and extreme way – and why he had been unable to fulfill the mourning process and eventually accept Tania's death.

And it is the same question that informs a strong critique of the very phenomenon of DID, which tends to overlap substantially with depression, PTSD, anxiety, depersonalization and derealization disorder,[26] bipolar disorder, and other labelled conditions. There are countless instances of trauma the world over – yet relatively few occurrences of DID. This conversive disorder is triggered or aggravated by a variety of traumatizing factors, but not necessarily by abuse in childhood, contrary to a controversial, partly politicized claim that was in fashion for some years and that yielded intense debates especially in the 1990s. In his epochal book *Rewriting the Soul: Multiple Personality and the Sciences of Memory*, published at the height of these debates in 1995, philosopher Ian Hacking addressed the issue in the light of attempts by the first scientific psychologists in the nineteenth century to understand memory as 'a surrogate for the one aspect of a human being that seemed resistant to science', that is, the soul, which until then had always pertained to metaphysics or religion. Hacking reminds us that Théodule Ribot, in the positivist spirit of the nineteenth century, had sought to establish a scientific law of forgetfulness that covered 'both forgetting caused by physical lesions, and forgetting caused by psychic shock' or what we would call trauma (the very law that Vanessa's amnesia did not seem to match).[27] In Ribot's time, multiple personalities 'seemed splendid for showing that a person was not constituted by a single transcendental, metaphysical or spiritual self or ego', since it was acceptable to say that there could be many people within one body.[28]

It is admittedly odd that one self could vanish, as it were, while another emerges. But then, we all contain multitudes – to paraphrase the oft-cited, parenthetical ('I am large, I contain multitudes') of Walt Whitman's 1892 'Song of Myself'. We are capable of expressing a thought that we promptly forget. Our tastes, needs, moods, looks, change over time, according to how we feel or who we are with. So will our concerns, passions, loves, political opinions – as William James had noted just two years before Whitman in his *Principles of Psychology*.[29] Rather than as a static *entity*, the self might be best viewed as a dynamic *process* of constantly updated body representations that begin early in life, aligned with the dynamic process that is autonoetic memory.[30] Forgetting, then, can be seen as a missing link in that process rather than a missing bit of the self. Louis had turned memory-making into an obstruction, the past into an ever-present presence. It was possible that his helplessness when faced with Tania's fatal illness had triggered an earlier instance of helplessness that had occurred in different circumstances and had led him early on to use a dissociative method to cope with everyday life, in a manner that for long had remained less explicit or visible, and that arose out of a child's rich imagination. His capacity to dissociate, following van der Kolk's description of a traumatic replay, would have then made him unable to 'surrender' to the sad reality, since he would have associated surrender with the 'paralysis' he may have experienced when she died, unable as he had been to do anything to save her. This stress response of the autonomic nervous system could well have fed into the deconstruction of his embodied sense of self, hence the loss of control over his own limbs. His body matrix may have been distorted by uncorrected 'bottom-up' prediction errors, his self now persisting not as a seamless, constantly updated whole but in parts, as a conflicted, optimistic-pessimistic dyad, made manifest in the diagonistic apraxia.[31] He could no longer move his limbs at will because his sense of bodily self-ownership was as askew as the integrity of his experiencing, autonoetic self. His agency, just as in the case of Geraldine or indeed Thomas, was dislocated, and dysfunctional – except for the fact that unbeknown to both his internal narrative voices, he was the author of his own splitting in two.

Louis was a more structured person than Thomas, and his cognitive abilities were intact, though like Jeanne, Caroline felt she was caring for a child. But his dissociation was a long-lasting phenomenon, while Thomas's inability to inhabit his own will seemed to be the manifestation of a somewhat shorter crisis that, according to clinical histories of cases like his, would resolve, probably for good. Louis was not in a state of crisis in that his split personality was itself an elaborate, nonconscious strategy to avert crisis. That was why the psychiatrist intuited that the clinician should bring the patient to a state of crisis in order to kickstart the process of reintegration. Both cases, however, showed us how labile our sense of self is, regardless of what may have brought Thomas and Louis to their respective, and admittedly very different, states of dissociation.

While most of us manage to maintain a sense of unity within our changing selves, most of the time, the complex processes at work that constitute the dynamic self, involving bodies, histories, narratives, and emotions, can break down. We take these processes for granted until something goes wrong. Even when all is right, and perhaps especially when we are feeling entire, and at peace with ourselves, we can suddenly catch sight of ourselves in between two mirrors, as I did as a child in the entrance hall of my parents' building, and wonder who or what is this self we see, show, share, and talk out. We are at once a corporeal, physical body that must survive and a living subject that exists in time, the one overlapping with the other – most of the time, because sometimes the unity dissolves.[32] Sometimes we can look at ourselves as if from the outside. Contemplation can turn into dissociation, for a few minutes, until we return to the here and now. If we are lucky, and a poet as my mother was, we can translate the feeling self into verse for the future. And even as we live the life we must or can live, we are each at once solid and fragile, centre and periphery, substance and predicate, transparent and opaque, simple and complex, one and many, alone and connected. Our self in time perhaps is but a thin gauze wrapped around the shifting elements we are made of.

9

The Affront

There is a pain—so utter—
It swallows substance up—
Then covers the Abyss with Trance—
So Memory can step
Around—across—upon it—
As one within a Swoon—
Goes safely—where an open eye—
Would drop him—Bone by Bone.

Emily Dickinson, F515 (1863)

The elements from which we are made are ancient. Each one of our experiences connects us to all that precedes us. I looked up at Mars the other night, which was shining alone in the Paris sky, unusually bright. It seemed close to Earth, as I breathed, quiet in the dark room, feeling happily insignificant – enjoying the freedom I have to contemplate planets and existence, the fabric of memory, what it has meant to be a daughter, and who my mother remains. To take the time to think about what is happening to her. About the course of my life, as time ticks on, as my children grow, so slowly and so fast. The earth rotates, so slowly and so fast. Mars is so close, and so far. We are and are not the measure of space, or time. I am trying to safeguard within myself all the childhood memories that come to mind, many of which I realize I have taken for granted, and may otherwise disappear as my mother's neurons die. It is already too late to retrieve some details. Recently I asked her – because I wanted to know if we still shared so strong a memory – if she remembered her recipe for the chocolate cake she used to make for our birthdays, and which I loved so much that birthdays became synonymous with chocolate cake for my whole childhood and even adolescence. She said 'oh yes of course, I remember the recipe' – then was about to continue, but immediately after had no idea what she was about to say. Of course she remembered. At least 'of course'. I suggested it may not have had flour. 'Flowers, you mean,' she retorted. 'Flowers! All cakes have flowers.'

The countdown to rejoining stardust begins with birth but we only start hearing the timer loud and clear when time is up for the person who nurtured us from infancy – indeed for the mother who gave birth to our time on earth, if we are lucky enough still to have our mother in adulthood. Many patients who came to the clinic had been running too fast to have leisure for Mars and metaphysics, and many had not bothered until then to listen to the timer. Most of the families of those with dementia had the time to realize what was happening, although many had difficulty accepting the painful reality. But other, younger patients were in the midst of their fast, full lives when a break happened that shocked them out of their planned trajectories. The complexity of the mechanisms at work within each person escapes most of us most of the time – and then it can go strangely wrong. Just as dementia usually appears progressively, as if playing hide-and-seek with our definitions of pathology until it gets tired of playing, so there are also sudden traumas that can cause a cognitive blight and debilitating disturbances, unexpectedly blocking the view to a future, stopping life in its tracks – without there being any apparent illness.

Greg is such a patient. He is in his early forties. He wears a gold chain and small round glasses, and seems energetic and affable as he enters and sits down. But he is not very well. We have learned from the anamnesis that he burned out at work, a few years after moving from the countryside, near the Loire valley, with his wife and their three children to the Paris suburbs. Here he had successfully set up a new business, building and insulating roofs, in association with a larger company of which it became a part. And then it happened quite fast – his body told him to stop, as he put it when he told us his story. He was working hard, over fifteen hours a day, at weekends too. Then one day, as he got out of his car, he suddenly felt dizzy, and lost consciousness, though he came to shortly after. He was perfectly aware of what had happened. And he paid little attention to the episode. He was allowed leave, but didn't take it. After that, though, the pressure increased at work. He received threatening letters, and then anonymous death threats by text message, about which the company president refused to do anything. The atmosphere worsened. And that last summer, as he arrived at work, he felt dizzy again, then nauseous, and then he vomited. His head felt heavy. As he tried to park, he nearly crashed his car into another one parked on his left. A colleague who was standing there said that he looked unwell, as if drunk, and should go home. He did, though he doesn't recall how he managed to drive back. His wife, whom he called, returned home from work, took one look at him, and called an ambulance. At the ER, a vascular episode was suspected, though the MRI performed in hospital showed nothing significant. He was prescribed aspirin.

That was the last day of his life before his life today, as he himself puts it to the doctors. From then on, he felt nothing on his whole left side, neither pain nor pleasure. It was numb. He had what is called a hypoesthesia of the left hemibody – a loss of sensation on the left side of his body.[1] And he had a visual deficiency as well: he would bump into objects that were in his left field of vision. But worse still, he had formed no new memories since that fatal day: he had anteretrograde amnesia. As far as he was concerned, Trump was still a businessman, and Macron was still minister of finance. He was stuck in time, somewhat like the famous HM. He kept track by writing notes on his phone. He got lost in his house. Yet he knew who he was, that he had children, what their names were. And he never asked the same question twice.

When the neurologist asks him if life is better now or then, he says it is just different. He can no longer work, but he can spend more time with his family, and that is good. He can't follow games with his kids, but at least he is there, though he is tired a lot of the time, and generally slowed down. He wants to recuperate his capacities, his energy, his sense of time – what used to take him five minutes takes him two hours now. His wife has to do everything. He can't work anymore. Sure, there are no more death threats, but he is in an odd place. When asked by the neurologist whether he is on official sick leave, he says the information is written on his phone. When asked to write numbers, he is unable to do so accurately, though he seems to know how to write the alphabet. When asked where he lives, and how he used to get to work, he is unable to respond. He has no idea where the main cities of France are. He knows he has forgotten much. He is vague about the amount of time he has been in hospital, though he doubts it is a matter of weeks. He knows the hospital is in Paris only because that, too, is written on his phone. And his attention is poor: he can watch cartoons with his children for a few minutes at most. He is not aware of their ages, of the sense of time passing. The spatiotemporal continuum of his life has collapsed. And the meanings of words elude him. Prompted, he can say what a stamp is, and an envelope, but not a kangaroo.

'What is the explanation for this change,' asks the neurologist, 'can you tell me?' Greg replies lucidly: 'My body said "stop", long after I should have done so, after I was first given sick leave. I didn't take it then, because pressures were too high at work, and I had to keep going anyway. But I should have stopped at that point.' He remembers the day the stop happened, the last day of his life before. He describes the unfolding of it all – the vertigo, nausea, car veering to left, ambulance. He has no recollection how long he stayed in hospital then, nor whether the visual issues started at the same time as the other ones. And he doesn't know whether he is still on leave, or, if he is, whether he is on full pay – that information is also on the phone. Of course his wife knows the information too – she had to stop work as well, to care for him. He does realize that he could not work again, not in his current state. He doesn't think of his new dependency as a problem. It is 'real life' for him. He does not feel lost in a life without landmarks, because he is aware of what he has, and of what happened.

Yes, he knows exactly what happened. As the psychiatrist takes over from the neurologist and prompts Greg for details about what got him to this point, a peculiar shift takes place. He begins to tell us an extremely detailed story. It comes out like a thriller. A generally malevolent atmosphere in the work-place. The death threats from another employee, sent by text message. The lackadaisical attitude of the boss, who hired a lawyer but washed his hands of any responsibility. The narrative he shares with the psychiatrist has nothing to do with the helpless picture of himself he was giving the neurologist just a few moments before. The contrast is staggering. But it is also clear that he was not feigning his feelings of helplessness earlier. Greg is truly incapacitated in his daily life. The phone- and wife-dependent existence he is conducting now is the direct result of an acute shock. Greg says he doesn't think about the death threats. 'We talked, I fixed it,' he says, faintly sounding like a mobster. 'They understood I was straight.' Straight enough to be broken by stress, it seems. The legal details tumble out of his mouth, even though he says his wife is the one who deals with the bureaucratic and financial aspects of the case. He says he has no desire to press charges, just to have the work accident recognized as such and to move on. He is perfectly aware of chronology and the issues at stake. He is suddenly an articulate expert, comes across as the man used to being in charge, the experienced working guy who has simply seen too much and washed his hands of responsibility. He attributes the nastiness of the working environment to the regional culture – Parisians are more brutal than people in the provinces, he says.

The psychiatrist asks Greg – as he asks most patients – if he is depressed. The only response is that he wakes up tired. He then resumes his story, fluently, engaged and passionate, still angry at times about the professional and psychological affront he suffered – from without, and then, from within. He speaks for nearly half an hour. After he leaves, the neurologist is clear: this is a case of somatoform conversion (another one). Greg has somatized his status as ill, and, not unlike Claire, remains stuck in a state of shock. But he is potentially as able as before. He can be helped. There is discussion amongst the clinicians of prescribing an anti-depressant to combat his lop-sided psychological inertia. He needs to get out of this strange twilight zone he has entered, and recuperate the spatiotemporal bearings he has lost.

How is it, I wonder as I listen, that one can lose one's spatio-temporal bearings at all? What are these bearings, exactly? How do we experience time, and why is it that our sense of it shifts according to our state of mind and state of health? We shape ourselves in time, and it may be that time escapes our conscious grasp when the brain's predictive processing, which allows for the constant transformation of past into present via the future, becomes dissociated from external clocks, and from the times of others. Amnesia, such as Vanessa's, but also such as my mother's, is exactly such an occurrence. Memory could be conceived as the neuronally encoded representation of perceived temporal units, a constant re-creation enacted in a perpetual present that biology transforms into an arrow, turning each individual into a repository of time, whose traces accumulate in the form of biological changes within our bodies and on our skin. Everything, including Mars, whether cosmic, geological, architectonic, artefactual or artistic, is situated within time. All of these age – but biological time is indexed on the uniquely biological properties of what is organically evolved. The sense of time is profoundly tied in to our own awareness of consciousness – the one necessitates the other – and is the most elusive of concepts, because it seems to be constantly passing, as if it were a spatially extended but unseizable element, water, fire, or air, flowing over, across, and within us earthbound creatures. This is an ancient puzzle that leads us into the realms of physics and cosmology, to the laws of thermodynamics, to questions about the direction of time, to distinctions between experience and ontology. But here, down on earth, Greg is experiencing an amnesia, that is, a temporal absence, very different from Vanessa's, though like hers a testament to how biologically (and, to follow Friston, computationally) encoded is our very capacity to make chronological sense of ourselves within the world.

It occurs to me now that this peculiar manifestation of human biology fits with Kantian metaphysics – and I haven't thought deeply about Kant since my days as a philosophy undergraduate. Kant had posited that space and time are the subjective, *a priori* conditions of experience – the very condition for there being any experience at all – and are not derived from experience *a posteriori*. We cannot know them in themselves but they shape all we can experience as an *a priori* intuition. We alone experience them by dint of our very ability to have subjective experience.[2] But is Kant right? We know that without the sense of temporality embedded within memory, there would be no unitary self, and many emotions dependent on representing what is not immediately present to the mind would not exist – hope, anxiety, regret, pride, sadness, joy, love, and indeed the guilt that my mother no longer feels. Yet change is embedded within the very current of a unitary, subjective life. We have that 'core self' I have been feeling is so strong in my mother – but unless or until a dementia dissolves the autobiographical self, we also develop throughout our lives, build an identity through a time that is also outside us: things age, and we age in time, all things relative to each other. Being is being in time, in each others' time. We change and experience time, in time, and especially in shared space and time.

Whatever happened to the experience of time in Greg's case, then? Metaphysics and biology do connect. And our biology may give us the key to the metaphysics. Where is Greg in time, exactly, and is there a Greg outside his time? Vanessa was firmly situated within her present, despite having lost a segment of her past. Greg is not in his present. He is not as radically lost as HM or Sekine, who could no longer acquire experience because their cerebral injuries had rendered them unable to encode new memories, but he is not in his life, either. At first glance, none of this makes much sense. Start with the assumption that if all is well, we awake each morning aware of being the person we were the day before. Personal identity seems, according to this standard view, to rely on temporal continuity, and the two, as John Locke had described in his *Essay Concerning Human Understanding*, in 1690, are deeply connected.[3] Of course, we also change – and this is what complicates the notion of personal identity. For Hume, writing a few decades later in the *Treatise of Human Nature*, 'man is a bundle or collection of different perceptions which succeed one another with an inconceivable rapidity and are in perpetual

flux and movement', and just as flux characterizes our experience, so it is inherent in our identity attributions, that is, in
our recognizing an entity as one despite its changing: a small
oak is the same tree as the grown oak, he writes, just as the
'infant becomes a man, and is sometimes fat, sometimes lean,
without any change in his identity.'[4] What binds the identity
together, the 'source of personal identity', is memory. 'Had we
no memory, we never should have any notion of causation, nor
consequently of that chain of causes and effects, which constitute our self or person.' By contrast, neurophilosopher Georg
Northoff (who used to claim to be a neo-Kantian), argues that
'memories are not the candidate for preserving the identity of
the person over time', since whatever is encoded is continuously
updated. Moreover, Northoff emphasizes 'the continuity of
change' as opposed to continuity despite change: 'the brain
shows continuous change and variability in its resting-state
activity'.[5] This may be a neurological key to the continuity of
a changing identity through time and causal and spatial structures. As it happens, Greg has a strong notion of causation.
And he does not doubt who he is. So something else, something
not imagined by Hume, has gone askew. Something not
mentioned by Northoff either. Something bodily.

Two hundred years after Hume, William James stated in his
chapter on 'The Perception of Time' in *The Principles of
Psychology* that duration is the key to our perception of time.
'It is only as parts of this duration-block that the relation of
succession of one end to the other is perceived . . . we seem
to feel the interval of time as a whole, with its two ends
embedded in it.'[6] Time flows, but it is made of moments that
we divide into units: 'we are constantly conscious of a certain
duration – the specious present – varying in length from a few
seconds to probably no more than a minute.' And this duration,
that which he calls 'specious present' (explicitly borrowing from
one E. R. Clay, the pseudonym of a philosopher named Robert

Kelly), 'is the original intuition of time'.[7] He surmises there is a 'fairly constant feature in the brain-process' that *must be the cause of our perceiving the fact of time at all* (his italics). The content of this duration 'is in a constant flux, events dawning into its forward end as fast as they fade out of its rearward one, and each of them changing its time-coefficient from "not yet", or "not quite yet", to "just gone", or "gone", as it passes by.' The recall of the event beyond this 'specious present', however, 'is an entirely different psychic fact from its direct perception in the specious present as a thing immediately past.'[8]

The experience of time in this account is separate from memory. Yet meaningful, longer-scale human experience is nothing without memory and imagination, which, as we saw earlier, recruit overlapping cerebral functions.[9] When we recollect a moment, we also imagine and reconfigure it within a new present. The notion of time Augustine develops in his *Confessions*, which figured as I was trying to puzzle out Vanessa's very different case, has at its centre the dependence of our notion of past and future on memory: our very psychology, and our very ability to understand causality, are an aspect of the metaphysics of time. The self is constructed along with the sense of a socially shared temporality which we acquire progressively during childhood – and so, since the self is embodied, our perception of time is, like all else, profoundly embodied too. A disruption in embodiment does bend the sense of time – and this has been shown experimentally.[10]

It is possible that Greg has stopped experiencing time – and that it corresponds to his feeling lost in space (in his own home) as well. He is stuck in a perpetual present despite the fact that there is no neurological damage rendering him unable to encode and consolidate new memories as was the case for HM. What he suffers is akin to what other patients with schizophrenia or depersonalization disorders experience: they feel detached from their bodies and their sense of time is distorted.[11] Just as Greg has lost sensation in one half of his body, so he has lost a dimension that is essential for experience to make sense. He knows that the narrative that led to this loss is solidly in place, but it is as if he is locked up in a dimension that is no longer his – a dimension to his left, where he nearly crashed the car, where he no longer feels himself to be. The Greg we see looks whole, and normally embodied, but his self-narrative is split, just as are his memory and his body: he half feels, half knows. The integrity of experience is split, and so no longer feels like his. He is as if displaced. Anyone who has had invasive surgery can testify to a similar experience: an assault on the physical integrity of the self is an assault on the self. There is no distinction between the one and the other. Nor is there much of a vocabulary to describe the feeling of decentring. The cognitive outcome of the affront Greg has suffered may be a more radical version of the interoceptive outcome of surgery. It is as if the trauma he has suffered had driven a surgical wedge into his whole raison d'être.

We all experience variations in how we experience time's passage: slow, fast, too slow, too fast. The Jamesian perception of duration can shift according to whether one reports it during or after the experience. It is only when we needn't think about it, when we are wholly engaged within an activity that takes our attention away from our embodied self, that it feels homeostatically just right, like the temperature of the small bear's porridge in *Goldilocks* – with no sense of 'lost' time or panic over 'too little' time. Conversely, duration is diluted when we pay attention to time passing and the clock ticking and are not engaged with an activity. Neurophysiology, including notably the dopaminergic system (the various pathways in the brain responsible for the processing of dopamine), modulates the perception of temporal duration and of the timing of intervals.[12] But this has only been tested on the sort of short timescale James had in mind with his 'specious present', as opposed to the longer-scale, existential dimensions, where time expands or shortens, leading to boredom or to a sense of 'running against time'.

But even these longer-scale dimensions are ultimately constituted by moments during which we are more or less present to, and aware of, our embodied processes. Our experiences of time and emotional processes are connected. Neuroscientist A. D. Craig, who has done seminal work on the neurobiological bases of interoceptive processes,[13] suggests that 'the neural substrates responsible for sentience across time are based on the neural representation of the physiological condition of the body.'[14] The very processes of interoception that represent our homeostatic condition 'constitute an image of the "material me" or the sentient self at the immediate moment of time.'[15] These processes, in his view, are possibly what ensures that we experience as a continuum 'subjective emotional awareness within a finite present'. Craig finds that these processes may also be related to the appreciation of music, which he describes as 'the rhythmic temporal progression of emotionally laden moments': emotional context and content both modulate temporal perception. Time expands when we queue or wait for a train – when the absence of distractions entrains a higher attention to our bodily states.

Over the years, heartbeat detection tasks have yielded more and more precise data regarding our interoceptive capacities, notably through experiments carried out and analysed by neuroscientist Sarah Garfinkel and her colleagues.[16] Heartbeats are, like any beat, timed. Accurate counting of heartbeats in relation to precisely timed sounds has been shown to correlate with activation of the right anterior insula, which is crucial in interoceptive processes, as Craig had first shown.[17] The heart–brain dialogue, it has been found, has a direct impact on temporal awareness.[18] We feel the variations in our physiologically given sense of time every day, our perceptions and our feelings or affective valence directly connected to the cardiac cycle of systole-diastole and to heart-rate variability, our emotions modulated in synchrony with cardiac rhythms.[19] Staying in tune with time is entwined with the body and with the ANS remaining within a viable homeostatic range as the central nervous system responds to interoceptive and exteroceptive inputs. The sense of self and the sense of time coalesce. Embodied time is subjective time. And it must be synchronous with the embodied time of others for the individual to make sense of time, to communicate and to comprehend the world's time. Inner time can only make sense in terms of outer time – and vice versa. We understand each other's rhythms in speech, laughter, dance, love. We enjoy drumbeats that mimic the heart's beat. When we are isolated in our internal time, duration is lost, days and nights grow into one unintelligible mass, as is so often the case in depression, for instance. It seems that the accuracy of time-duration detection falls away in psychiatric pathologies.[20] The squeezing, stretching, knotting, dissolving of time is inherent in all states of ill health, or even mild unease, and in all moments of emotional transition. Dislocation from the ordinary spatiotemporal continuum is an aspect of dislocation from the social continuum.

It has also been suggested – by Karl Friston and neuroscientist Gyorgy Buszáki – that our sense of a continuum, which is at the core of our subjective experience, may be independent of the actual succession of events.[21] Our concepts of duration, such as fast and slow, do not tell us about the content of the event. Succession is separate from the events that succeed each other, and this distinction may apply to the sequential aspect of our experience – to our sense of a self-narrative, as it translates, notably, into episodic memory. The hippocampus is the structure that processes temporal succession in the form of memory, and it is distinct from the neocortex, which encodes the content. *When* and *where* are not the same as *what*. Sequences differ from any specific content. This is how the brain 'approximates' the world, and eventually creates meanings out of this faculty – hence Greg's strange experience of having interrupted time: the *what* of his life is no longer temporally situated. Friston and Buszáki note how 'the order of words during reading (but not listening) depends on where I am looking' so that, in a sense, location is 'a special case of temporal organisation'. The distinction, they write, is 'analogous to the role of a librarian (hippocampus, pointing to the items) in a library (neocortex, where semantic knowledge is stored). The organized access (in spatiotemporal trajectories) to neocortical representations (what) then becomes episodic information.' I see this with my mother, who recalls the *what*, but not the *when* and *where*, her self-narrative wholly unbound. It is helpful to picture her mind in this way – a lot of *whats* unmoored from time and place, losing their meaning, and their relevance.

Another, related account given by Buzsáki with neuroscientist Rodolfo Llinás[22] reminds us that 'navigation and memory are deeply connected,'[23] which would explain why Greg gets lost in his home, and perhaps also why my mother sometimes thinks her flat is a hotel. Both navigation and memory involve the hippocampus and its interface with the neocortex, the entorhinal cortex, set within the medial temporal lobe. And the hippocampus is active in interoceptive processes.[24] Episodic recall, including recall of embodied, multimodal experiences, involves a projection back in space and time, while we travel into the future through prediction. We navigate space and time.[25] We create internal meanings out of encounters in the environment, and the combination of what, where, when structures our embodied position within time, and constitutes our episodic memories. We connect events and create the order out of which we create meaning,[26] but damage to the hippocampus creates an inability to process the order of events.

This is exactly what happens in Alzheimer's. It is helpful to think of the hippocampus and entorhinal cortex when I see my mother. But they are not the whole story.

Greg does not have a damaged hippocampus, but the complex navigational function we need to live daily life has been as if disabled. He is a ship unable to sail, stuck in the sand. He has thrown meaning and meaningfulness overboard. He has to wait out this period of his life, on the shore – giving time to time, as many doctors often like to say, ultimately conceding that time is the only tool they have, though it isn't theirs to use. Confined at home and without a job, without purpose or orientation towards the future, Greg would have passed for a melancholic in the days of humoural medicine, in need of light, exercise, a sleep regimen and a calibrated diet. Such existential torpor would have been holistically addressed, which may, or may not have worked. We have a more precise understanding of the causes of his state today, but the clinicians have few new instruments available to them with the exception of carefully calibrated pills. They may help, regardless of their pharmacological heft, because he does want to return to time, and recuperate the memory that it has swallowed, like Chronos devouring his children. Swallowing these pills day after day may remind him of inner and outer daily rhythms, of his competent wife and growing children, and of the world out there that had grown so full of danger and violence, but has now become more acceptable. His self had turned out to be so much less impervious to the world's impacts than he had thought – he the man who built roofs and insulated them against heat, chills and tempest. He has insulated himself against the world and time since they struck him down, but there is no life in a perpetual present, and he knows that. He wants to catch up, get up from under his protective roof, sail off. And unlike many patients who come into this room, he can: he has time and life ahead of him.

When I was a child, like most children I measured years in birthdays – and in the twice-yearly occurrence of the birthday cake, one for Alba, one for me, at six-month intervals. The passing of time was otherwise a vague reality, until the end of one school year when I suddenly realized that *it would never be so again*: that class, that teacher, that set of children had been a one-off, and the goodbye as we left for our Middle-Eastern summer was forever. I was about eight when the unbearable realization hit. It was always the time of swallows in Paris, late June with its light and colour, the longest days, and the wrenching melancholy of their cries, deep into the endless evening. It dawned on me then that the childish scale of time was all wrong. That duration was a far larger matter, beyond my life, and that the swallows' cries were like its heartbeat. I looked up at the sky where they flew, into the northern blue. I decided I would be an astronomer. (I later gave up on the idea when I realized I would have to be good at maths, which I wasn't. But I kept the books and I recently gave one of them to my sons.)

I still associate the promise of summer with the bittersweet sound of swallows' cries. Summer is my season, when everything stops, growth is at its apex, the timer goes quiet. Then the school year starts again, the days shorten. The timer ticks again, always faster, louder. Time contracts with each autumn, though by now the summers have started shrinking as well. The physics of time and space are a consolation for the biology that constrains us within our lifespan and can condemn us to confusion. Mars is a calming sight. My mother no longer has a sense of time and so she is calm, mostly, unless contradicted or forced into an action she has no wish to execute. Hers is a specious present, multiplied over and over. Meaning within is dissolving, but at least she knows a cake has flowers. I am holding on. I am here, now, and I remember. Meaning has never been so clear. I still have time and life ahead of me.

10

Coda

while we close a door
flocks of birds are flying through winters
of endless light

W. S. Merwin, from 'At the Same Time',
in *Poetry* (December 1970)

Consciousness and its twists and turns, despair, hope, sometimes humour in the face of the dislocations of self, memory,
words and limbs – the human person observing itself as other,
or as self: all these were present during the sessions at the
hospital. Each of us can experience how manifold is our self.
We are here to make sense of the world, and of each other,
but things do not always make sense, and everyone's capacities
fluctuate, from day to day, even hour to hour. One may awake
having understood the mysteries of the universe, and only be
able to think of the dinner menu come evening. Our bodily
states are constantly adjusting, our perceptions, emotions,
sensations constantly calibrated and calibrating whatever the
organism needs most urgently to attend to. From Mars to
chocolate cake. At best. This is also why the border between
normal and pathological can be very unclear.

Still, as I know first hand now, there are states of disintegration at the very end of the scale. Pathology can jump at you
like a beast from the shadows. I did not see any psychiatric

patients at their worst. But many patients who came into the hospital room presented with symptoms that signalled incipient neurodegeneration – and I was unaware at the time that they echoed my mother's own confusion. Two such patients figure here, but I chose early on not to dwell on the others, one of whom was a woman diagnosed, by the end of the clinical session, with frontotemporal dementia, or FTD. She had been an accountant but was no longer able to count. She stated that dogs had three legs, forgot words, names of films, the names of her grandsons. She had depression, had disinhibitedly appeared naked in public, ate voraciously, was spatially disorientated and aggressive, and she was apathetic – that is, she had a debilitating lack of motivation. Her decision-making no longer functioned effectively and so her emotional memory wasn't maintained either, and she was unable to elaborate on her emotional states. Her grasp of semantics and meaning had become fragile, and she associated words figuratively– hence the three-legged dog. The clinical eye of one of the neurologists, who sometimes seemed to me to be akin to a living MRI scanner, pointed to orbito-frontal lesions that would have accounted for the attentional issue and the unravelling of willed action and social interaction.[1] The actual MRI had shown no focal lesion, and no hypometabolism in the frontal lobe. Yet as ever, the clinic trumped the imaging, and as ever, the doctor was capable of the sort of insight that a machine does not have: this, the neurologist said, was certainly an insidious evolution of fronto-temporal and lateral lobe degeneration, a fragmentation of the organs of semantic knowledge, like the breaking up of a highway node, as he put it, into a state of psychotic delirium, a 'paraphrenia' (*pará*, besides and *phrene*, mind).[2] What we were witnessing was a devastation. When her husband mentioned she seemed a little better than she had been over the past year, he was actually witnessing in her disinhibition – her uncontrolled but lively impulses – the other side of the terrible indifference that comes with apathy, since both are symptoms of neurological damage. It was like a wave overtaking a dyke. Eventually, explained the neurologist after the couple had left, the apathy would win out. He mentioned a frontal patient he had seen who, six years into his illness, suddenly returned to being his functioning self – one blessed day. Then he returned to his apathic state.

The clinical analysis was fascinating in what it revealed about our self-understanding, and about the complexity of the cerebral processes that get derailed when the frontal lobe, struck by one of those various kinds of proteinopathies, stops working as it normally should. But I decided not to set down her case here in any detail, because her visit was harrowing to witness, the suffering of her husband matched by her own disarming anosognosia. It was after seeing her that my initial thought of centering this whole book on anosognosia – and on that state as defining of the human condition – struck me as too lighthearted: there are levels of unknowing, together with levels of suffering, such that the comedy of ordinary neurosis cannot apply. And yet, even in this hopeless case, the person, though unable to reflect and know herself for what she was, remained present, enjoying the session, curious, still alive. We do not let go so easily – just as consciousness will not dissolve so fast, either. And it is so with my mother as well. We know where she is heading, yet there remains joy in her, and in our interactions. There is presence, and life. The fact that she is surrounded by the sort of care I could not provide without distress on any side does help a great deal. This was not always the case for all patients, many of whom were already or would end up in so-called care homes. The logistics of caring for patients afflicted with neurodegeneration are not the stuff of comedy either.

And so, I returned to what got me started in the first place, however banal the thought: the fact that we can understand anything at all about the brain, armed with the brain to do so, is astounding. Just as astounding is the complexity inherent in higher cognition, in our capacity to manipulate ideas and thoughts, and causally and spatiotemporally to situate ourselves. I cannot help but wonder how we ever create meaning and make sense, how it is we are able to hold it all together, most of the time, so well that we can invent stories and create meaning in the first place. The embodied mind is what imagines, thinks, feels, and also what projects, conceptualizes, defines. Even when it ceases to appraise new data, or when the cells that encode memories turn into tombstones. The material and necessarily imagined immaterial me are one. Yes, take that, René, and it is I the grown human being saying so, not the dog pictured on my mother's apron. This feat of understanding is unlikely, in a way, and yet necessary given humanity's advanced capacities for metarepresentation, that is, our ability to study and represent the contents of our own minds – like a camera photographing itself, a mirror reflecting itself into another mirror, light shining upon light.[3]

When something goes wrong with the human mind or brain – the distinction between mind and brain remains, given that the brain serves the body and that the mind is not reducible to the brain – it becomes rather like the camera lens obscured, an oxydized mirror, light shining upon shade. Contrasts emerge, through the glass darkly. And the very fact that we easily use artefactual or technological similes to talk about our self-knowledge shows just how much we feel the need to separate ourselves from the object of study to study it at all – but also how misguided this is in the case of the embodied brain, which is remarkable precisely for its fabricating (for want of another word) our irreducible, corporeal subjectivity. This subjectivity can be illuminated by clinical acumen and scientific insight, but it cannot be abstracted into cases or into neuroscientific theories. Siri Hustvedt has noted in her essay 'The Delusions of Certainty' how Darwin never used machine metaphors to discuss evolution. Evolved, plastic, bloody, and embedded within humoural bodies and a complex world, brains have nothing to do with the 'dry' technologies our species have devised.[4]

And nowhere is this more apparent than in the clinic, where – despite the important addition of imaging – nomenclature, nosology, diagnostic practice, and clinical methodologies remain closer to their nineteenth-century roots than to any of the brave new world of science that is indeed producing the technology so many people are afraid will upend our humanity. Hustvedt spends many pages in her essay discussing and taking down this technological, 'post-human' fantasy. And indeed, looking at my mother, or indeed at a fragile patient, and at the paucity of effective cures, one is struck at how our biological nature, at once resilient and frail, is far more complex than any shiny instrument we could ever invent. We are organic beings, and cannot fully master our multiple selves. Imaging just confirms this: it helps us read into the complexity, but it doesn't constitute insight. All the technologies we are developing to see and act upon the world beneath the skin necessitate knowledge of a biological world that has not remotely yielded all its secrets – and it is arguable that, constituted of open systems as it is, as opposed to the deterministic world of physics, it will not ever do so.[5] Our understanding of what can go wrong with normal functioning is limited enough, though it is progressing, as we continue to define and redefine how we do normally function, and how, as Damasio has shown and the scientists working in his vein are showing with ever more precision, our sophisticated thought processes are on a tight continuum with feeling and the origins of life. We are biological through and through – and *bios*, in ancient Greek, means the course of a human life.

◆

When there is damage to the frontal lobe, as there was in the case of the woman I described here but to whose case I did not devote a chapter, directed attention no longer operates, apathy and abulia set in, appetites fire unhinged and unchecked.[6] But memories, feelings, the meaning of a life do not disintegrate at the same time. We have many layers and many parts. Structurally, the frontal lobe is adjacent to the primary motor and premotor cortexes, superimposed on all other parts of the brain, and is connected to the limbic system onto which projects the anterior insula. The insula, as Craig had first shown and as has been further seen in countless studies since then, is the part of the cortex so central to the interoceptive awareness which partakes in constituting the self.[7] It is hidden away within the lateral sulcus (the names of brain areas sometimes sound like the names of places on the moon) that separates frontal and parietal lobes from the temporal lobe. However, the insula has been shown not to be necessary for feeling: the cerebral processes involved are, as ever, more complex than would warrant any reductively locationalist, 'phrenological' temptation to assign to a specific mental function a precise location in the brain. In the same way, the ability to infer the location of cerebral damage from clinical signs may give the mistaken impression of simple one-to-one correspondences.[8] In fact our brains are made up of highly intricate, inter-related functions.

The narrative coherence that depends on these inter-related functions and that we attribute to our self-in-time is often considered to be what makes our lives meaningful: we need to envisage our lives as somewhat coherent, though always chaotic stories, with a beginning, middle and end all connected. Damage to autobiographical memory is devastating for this reason, and Vanessa suffered from its partial loss, of which she was aware. In the case of my mother, anosognosia ensures this is not so much a terrible experience as a progression into a new state – a process. We need to place ourselves within time, just as the brain itself fabricates our present as a prediction of the future based on past inputs. We saw it with Greg, and with other patients – when the coherence of the self is in jeopardy, there is also a dislocation from temporality. Of course, one may also argue against the idea that a meaningful life must be story-like, and attribute this need for coherence to a specific culture such as our modern Western one that values self-fulfillment and self-aware biographical progression. Philosopher Galen Strawson has argued that this sort of 'narrativity' is not necessary for our life to have meaning.[9] Meaning needn't be constructed out of chronology. We do not need to attribute a narrative coherence to our sense of temporality – even without it we are involved in the perpetual creation of a present.[10] There is no need to think of oneself as a character in a *Bildungsroman*. Without narrativity, one can still draw substantive connections between how elements in the past might manifest themselves in the present – as any basic psychological, not to say psychoanalytical view of the self would require – but 'the key explanatory linkings in psychotherapy are often piecemeal in nature,' as Strawson writes, and need not be overarching in a way that would be misleadingly generalizing.

Time, in other words, need not be modelled *post hoc* by a literary imagination for us to be able to grasp ourselves within it as a coherent whole. Narrativity might even breed a host of instances of self-deception, for instance a belief that to be 'true to oneself' one must think of oneself as being a certain type of person, and act in accordance with that coherent self-representation, interpreting all past actions and relationships and envisaging all future ones on that basis. Our inner coherence as a self, however constructed that identity, need not be bound to temporality in a metaphysical sense – Hume's problem with the continuity of identity, which he solved so radically, may indeed have been a false one in the first place.[11]

And this thought may be liberating. Time is strange enough, and the self enough of an enigma, not to have to link the two in a causal sense. But then narrativity contains chaos. It shapes the self as an entity belonging with other selves. Shared memories are the stuff of love. The flowers in the cake. A memory borne alone grows cold and sad. There is narrative because we cannot survive for long on our own. Our very cultures are narratives. And the stories I want to retrieve from my mother's ailing brain are a part of my culture. Even a theory is a story, if it is to hold together. The grammars of languages, and verbal meaning itself as well.

The passing of time – and the stories we live, even those we tell ourselves – is felt in the bones and seen on the skin. Ideally, growing old should be about growing serene at the notion of one's non-existence, and of the passage of time stopping for the embodied self that we each are. Death is the liminal border of our present, of our being-in-time: finality is the condition of our awareness of time unfolding – time itself is indeed not objective, as Augustine saw. When I was a child I was terrified of snakes, often imagining them writhing at the foot of my bed and making me unable to get up, for minutes at a time. This might have been an instance of a fear of change itself: each change is also a death. Asclepius, the Greek god of medicine, is always depicted holding a rod around which is coiled a snake: as an animal that periodically sheds and regrows its skin, the snake embodies change, therefore fertility, as well as death of course, which is the ultimate metamorphosis. Change itself is less frightening if one does not think of one's life in narrative terms – but doing so requires an inner freedom, indeed an ability to admire the perfected freedom of movement embodied by a moving snake. Change is inherent in all life. Neuronal activity is change. Homeostasis and allostasis are dynamic processes. Affect regulation happens constantly. Thoughts are not still. Indeed, as philosopher John Dupré suggests, one should think of life, and the self, and all relations, as processes, rather than entities.[12]

Illness is a process too. I see my mother slowly, progressively, lose her spatiotemporal bearings – not as Greg did, radically and temporarily, but permanently, her life losing its contours, movement no longer so free, the end of time constraining and twisting the meanings accrued during the long present that is a well-lived life. If the slips, confusions, messiness of neural degeneration[13] can be infuriating at first for the close of kin, this is because the person remains the same, wobbly at times but seemingly untouched. How does one relate to someone close who does not know she doesn't know? The bearings of our relationship certainly have been redrawn. Sometimes, though seldom now, a semblance of coherence returns for a few seconds, allowing me, very briefly, to relax back into normalcy until the next factual somersault, which then appears out of the damaged corner I had been trying to forget. By the time I had finished writing what turned out to be an intermediate version of this book – but felt like the final one – her grasp on space and time had become so tenuous that linear conversation was near impossible. She congratulated me when I told her I had finally finished: she still has a sense of conversational appropriateness, however generic it has become. 'I am so happy,' she said. I can gratefully hold on to that.

I also told her the book was partly about her. Maybe she understood this, briefly. I have written about her to honour what she has been, because she can no longer put herself on the page as she did so beautifully throughout her life as a writer. Neither a report of her brain scans nor her anamnesis as a patient would be of any use in conveying how baffling is the experience of dementia to those who witness it from up close, so I omitted those. The impartial observer in the room has become the partial daughter, the one informing the other. But what I have learned from observing and listening to the doctors certainly helps me better to accept, somehow, my mother's plight. If anything, they have taught me about empathy, and humility.

It will take much more study of the cerebral circuitry and cellular operations involved in the complex function that is episodic memory to help understand what exactly is being jumbled and lost. And also, to understand what remains. It is not surprising that neurodegeneration affects interoceptive ability,[14] since metacognition – our awareness of being aware – is deeply connected to interoception. It is possible that the disruption in the feedback that updates internal predictions, so crucial for the construction of subjective feeling states, affects the behaviour of patients with neurodegeneration, in particular those with Alzheimer's (or something akin to it) such as my mother, or those with FTD like the woman whose story I chose not to tell at length.[15] These novel findings could be applied to the clinic. And some of the experiments that are yielding them do depend on the presence in the study cohort of individuals presenting with a pathology. The work in neuroscience and psychology that is the background and foundation of the preceding pages does help explain how deeply embedded in physiology is experience in all its spatiotemporal, sensorial, emotive and cognitive dimensions. How emotions shape posture and how posture can determine intentions. But unless a theorist explicitly trains in a therapeutic practice in order to work translationally, finding out how we function is not the same as helping someone function.

Clinicians will send patients who may benefit to physical therapists whose job it is to understand the body–mind, as they explore muscles and bones under the skin, attentive to proprioceptive processes, able also to have an effect on interoceptive ones. But those therapies do not require medical degrees, any more than does the most refined yoga teacher, however aware of the relation between posture and emotion that teacher may be. The medical profession doesn't naturally allow for the sort of thinking that enables connections to be made between systems and organs that are not normally studied together. The brain–heart, brain–gut axes may be amongst the most promising and potentially transformative areas in neuroscience and the neuromedical fields, but it will be a while before their findings trickle down from lab to medical school to hospital.[16] And arguably, the trickle needs to grow into a stream. Individual disease and social unease are deeply connected. Regardless of our state of health, which is never perfect, we live as individual bodies within a collective body. And when diseases strike our brain, in particular, we depend on a collective will to catch us lest, or while we fall.

Doctors, though, are rarely in the position to take on board the latest theories such as those I have referred to throughout this book. It is hard to apply in practice even the best theoretical models, such as predictive processing, whose mathematics are as removed from the daily life of a patient as they are from the motions of waves on a beach. A scientific theory, like a narrative or story, or like known histories or myths, is a provisional construction: by definition it cannot encapsulate the complex, multilayered reality it is attempting to describe, recount or explain, and which will always escape our grasp. Events can never be predicted with certainty and narrative continuity as they are lived. How we represent our lives to ourselves is a constant construction whose meaning is in the construction – just as the dreams we remember are those to which we have attributed the narrative thread we seek to grab. The act of representation is itself the representation.

I realize what a privilege it was to sit in silently on the clinical sessions – so far removed from the theoretical models I had read about, and that I have used here to understand better what I saw there. I was neither the doctor called on to diagnose and offer help, nor the patient in pain or distress – nor yet at the time the patient's family. But all along, I knew, as most of us do most of the time, that fragility lurks around the corner, that no one is exempt from loss. This is why, even though I am an outsider to medicine and science, I am convinced that the medical and scientific professions, capable as they each are of helping to alleviate pain and giving us magnificent insight, rank at their best only when they forgo the temptation of mechanistic categorization that can magnify pain, and negate our nature and our humanity. Because our theoretical constructions can easily collapse before our mortal vulnerability, before our disordered biology, before the admirable attempt of each organism to keep track, adjust, correct, catch up just in the nick of time with the physical universe we were born into – until it no longer does. The biology is as fraught as it is mind-bogglingly miraculous to us self-contemplators. The narrative can fizzle out, the seeming temporality of a lived life can give way to the simple, timeless present of a beating heart, of thoughts and emotions known and unknown. This vulnerability is at the heart of the stories, even the scientific stories, we try to tell each other, and ourselves.

It is as a mother, who must always be at once vulnerable and strong, that I contemplate the rapidly growing children my own mother still recognizes, but will not see into their adolescence. They know what is happening. Just as they know I have been writing a book 'about the brain', so they know that their grandmother's state is 'about the brain'. They accept it. I think I accept it, but only by holding on within myself to who she has been since my childhood: the mother who baked that chocolate cake; the wife of the intense painter, who let him paint and draw her so many times; the sensitive poet whose words live under my skin. Just as those of us who have children never stop being parents, whatever that may mean, so no one ever stops being a son or daughter. We are not just born of others: humans remain vulnerable children for an exceptionally long time. It is during the early years that we acquire the capacity to forge bonds, to live in trust – to accept our basic vulnerability and build a life out of it, not despite it. And so it is in relation to our begetters – they or whoever or whatever in our life will stand for them – that we remain vulnerable. My mother embraced her vulnerability. That is precisely what poets do. This is why she still radiates a warmth that made her for years the soul of the parties I threw. Petite, curious, cracking jokes and always ready to listen, distressed at the distress of others, joyful with their joy, always tearful when moved. Young forever. And yet, not. Now she can no longer come to parties. But she still cares about her looks. She is helped into clothes and made up for the day. She has her hair coloured. She continues to see herself as she wishes others to see her. Appearances do matter. The mirror matters. Awareness of how we look partakes of self-awareness, and it can survive from within the depths of anosognosia.

I am standing between the two mirrors in my parents' building in Paris: the movements of my limbs are reflected into an infinitely multiplied choreography as I move and stretch my neck to try to see past myself to the shrinking image in the far distance. I alone experienced the vertiginous vision. I alone remember the feeling of seeing it back then, as the vulnerable child that I was who wanted to study stars and galaxies, and instead, once grown up, would study the embodied mind that is equipped to look at stars and galaxies – and at itself. I don't remember telling my parents about the multiple reflection when I reached the flat on the seventh floor. One day soon there will be no one there. Let there be sadness then. But I am not alone. I am just one of many. We are each one, and many.

Postscript

One's story—whose? does it matter?
one's gets set
in meters composed
of the years that lived with their narrator
till presto then largo they finally burst
the self's glued envelope.
I hear their cries compact the air.

> Anne Atik, from *Music on the Winter Solstice:*
> *Three Movements*, III published in *The American*
> *Poetry Review* (September/October 1997)

And now there is no one there.

My mother has joined my father at the Cimetière du Montparnasse. We all imagined, and feared, that she would simply continue unravelling. But a few weeks after this book was accepted for publication, all of a sudden she became very frail: the illness was affecting her motor system. Shortly after, unstable on her legs, unable to walk or get up on her own, she fell off her bed and hurt herself. From the hospital, as she awaited her X-ray, one of the marvellous women who cared for her videocalled me so that I could greet her. She asked her, 'What are you thinking about?' My mother responded, as promptly as she ever had: 'Do I look like I'm thinking?' Her humour was as tenacious as her illness. I was impressed, and happy, that she could make light even of that unpleasant situation.

It turned out she had broken her knee. She returned home with a massive cast on her right leg – the first cast of her life. She seemed nonplussed – but a little dazed. Ten days later, comfortably ensconced in her bed, she slept her way into unconsciousness, and peacefully died the next morning. A graceful exit just as the going was getting tough. She knew the party was ending, and slipped away, as if unwilling to be a burden, sparing herself and us the worst that was to come. I had wished her to leave gently in this way, in her home of fifty years and in her sleep, while her life still had meaning, while she still felt joy, and still recognized us. Perhaps she knew this and trusted me to let her go. The week before, when I last saw her awake, we had exchanged intensely loving good-byes – as if sensing it was the end. I had then got up to leave her side, with the usual 'I have to go,' to which she responded, 'Go ahead – go about living!' These were the last words of hers that I wrote down. Go about living.

My mother spent her last years in a state of total confusion mixed with total lucidity that was a kind of freedom, a solution to poetic striving and conceptual barriers, and all in the key of amusement. One can only be grateful for that, as this is not the experience of all Alzheimer's patients. I think she enjoyed the wild ride – she repeatedly said how happy she was. It was probably a relief, too, that at last there was nothing to be anxious or guilty about, and that her daughters stopped arguing with her. She spent most of her last months listening to music. When she interacted, always with love, recognition and gratitude, gems came out of her deepest mind. But it was difficult for those around her, as it always is.

Now she is gone, and mourning can be completed. A mother is the very condition of her children's existence, and the ultimate separation is life changing. It is akin to birth itself. The raw quality of physical separation – the immediate pain that inheres in losing a mother – reveals yet again what she was to me, and indeed that a mother is primarily to the child as *body*, as skin, as touch, as voice, as smell, as smile, as laughter, as gaze. It is lucky that she never ceased to recognize us, that there was still a twinkle in her eye when she beheld or heard me. And she did tell me to stop fussing with my hair a short time before dying, as always – what a relief that was. No matter the cognitive confusion, or how little she understood of ordinary conversation, my sister and I remained her precious daughters as long as she lived.

Her departure makes me realize even more strikingly than I knew how much of her self had remained despite the illness, but also that the time of illness had overshadowed much of what she had been before. The present always feels absolute, until it is no longer, and it can lead us to forget the texture of the past. The pages about her here are in a present that has suddenly stopped. With her existence now in hindsight, all that she had lost over these years is returning with renewed freshness. For she had a long, rich life. For fifty-nine years, it had been shaped by her intense, overbearing husband, whose presence continued to hover beyond his own death in 2010, his intensity such that he was as if embedded within the walls of our childhood flat – his art, and the portraits of her, illuminating its walls, his studio still full of his creative fervour, his books and desk unmoved. But she also had liberated herself after he died, writing, cultivating her friendships, forging new ones with writers many of whom are younger than me, and whom she continued inspiring until her last. She left her mark on everyone she ever met.

As I write these last lines, we are about to embark on rediscovering her past and writings. There is that memoir to retrieve – never completed, although her lifetime is now complete. The apartment on the seventh floor will soon be emptied – rich decades of life, art and learning moved and sifted, much of it to be preserved in our care and curation. Our parents had existed within its walls, but now their stories, and their creations, are a part of the wider world, perpetuating their presence. They are our heritage, and they also belong to a long, broad history.

Anne Atik was a great woman. Until her illness, as daughters we had often expressed annoyance with her anxiety, and at times felt frustrated – rather than just inspired as others were – by her rarefied world of poetry and aesthetics, because she was often bemused by ordinary practicalities. But such are mothers and daughters. The love we had for each other was immense. She was maternal to the core, utterly giving, utterly feeling – often tearful, often so very funny, and always true. We spoke every day, sometimes many times a day – as I did with my father too. We shared thoughts, writings, feelings. We wrote emails to each other. That all stopped with the illness. But until the very end she remained a youthful woman, attuned to the motions in those around her and to the flutters of the world – as if perpetually new to it. Even her dementia ended up helping me understand others, as well as myself, and my relation to her. Even in illness, she gave, laughed, and spread light.

Acknowledgements

I owe thanks to many people.

To Sarah Caro, my editor at Basic Books UK, who immediately embraced the finished manuscript, understanding it in a way writers can only dream of being understood, championing it and accompanying it to publication with dedication and immense care. She improved the text with subtle editing, as did Eric Henney at Basic Books US, who preceded Emma Berry and Caroline Westmore in welcoming and nurturing it warmly in turn. Candida Brazil's thorough and sharp-eyed copyediting much helped to tighten and clarify the text.

To Andrew Gordon, for taking it on and believing in it, and in the future. To Carrie Kania, who supported this project in its preliminary stages and without whom I may have given up early on. To Wendy Goldman Rohm, who provided the tough editorial advice I needed to rewrite the first draft. To Fran Bigman, who made invaluable comments on the second draft, showing me how I could turn this book into what it needed to be.

To Nigel Warburton, for providing me as editor at *Aeon* with the perfect forum through which to conduct investigations and develop key ideas, in particular for the article 'The Interoceptive Turn', published in June 2019, the research for which was central to the development of this book. To Kelly Burdick, executive editor at *Lapham's Quarterly*, and Lewis

Lapham, for commissioning two essays that have informed some of the pages here.

To the doctors who opened the door of the clinic at the Pitié-Salpêtrière hospital, for allowing me access to the consultations with the patients they received there, and giving me the green light early on to continue writing about what I saw and heard – they must remain anonymous to protect patients' privacy. And to those anonymous patients, whose lives and struggles taught me so much.

To the clinicians and researchers who, sometimes unbeknownst to them, have taught me a lot over the past few years. In alphabetical order: Guilhem Carle, for helpful insights about functional ailments from the psychiatric front. Quassim Cassam, for inviting me to a thought-provoking workshop on epistemic vices in modern medicine. Laurent Cohen, for sharing his neurological expertise especially about language, and for reading these pages. Martin Conway, for clues into navigating memory research. The, sadly, late biophysicist Maxime Dahan, for an unforgettable conversation about optogenetics, and his successor, Mathieu Coppey, with whom the conversation continued, about complex systems, cells and organisms. Richard Frackowiak, for provocative conversations about science and art. Sarah Garfinkel, for her important research on interoception and her contagious passion. Julie Grèzes, for clarifying exchanges about emotions. Patrick Haggard for his fascinating research on agency and for fruitful talks, Giandomenico Iannetti for his on pain and perception – both of their work made me realize that neuroscience at its best can be as aesthetic as art. Richard Lévy, for his support and for conveying his vast knowledge of neurology so clearly. Ann Lohof, for reading the first draft and telling me about her research on the cerebellum. Lara Migliaccio, for an informative conversation about dementias.

Gretty Mirdal, for bridging sciences and humanities at the Institut d'études avancées in Paris, where she has hosted inspiring conferences that helped me develop my ideas. Daniel Mograbi, for rich, transatlantic conversations about anosognosia. Lionel Naccache for encouraging me from the start and periodically enquiring as to how the book was going whenever we crossed paths on the hospital campus. Andreas Roepstorff, for stimulating exchanges, and helping to forge connections. Bill Sherman, for fostering the dialogue between psychology and the humanities at the Warburg Institute, whose mission still shapes my thinking, and for welcoming me back into its fold as Associate Fellow. David Sulzer, for conversations about dopamine and the history of its research. Catherine Tallon-Baudry, for sharing her research on interoception. Frédérique de Vignemont, for showing how philosophy and science can most fruitfully interact.

To the friends old and new who have nourished the writing, some of whom also read the work-in-progress - psychologists, neuroscientists, philosophers, social scientists, historians, clinicians, sundry writers.

First, the treasured dedicatees, who sustain me hugely, whose own work informs this book, and who know what WoW stands for. They are, alphabetically: Anna Ciaunica, for daringly and creatively bridging philosophy, science, and feminism. Katerina Fotopoulou, for joyously daring challenges, fiery insights, stirring lucidity and innovative work on the self in all its incarnations – and for her incisive comments on the first chapter. Vittorio Gallese, for his wise humanism and free-range passions, and for his necessary ideas. Siri Hustvedt, invaluable interlocutor, for her writing what she writes, for our potentially endless talk about minds, science, art, and more, for keeping me on track and on my toes – and for having read each draft, providing essential comments and encouragement at each stage. Mériam

Korichi, for metaphysical provocations, for her complicity, her optimism, and for inventing new worlds. Always and as ever, Gloria Origgi, the essential, vital force at my side, thanks to whom the best of life happens, from big ideas to big meals, and in whose generous company I began writing these pages during a Sicilian summer – and for reading and commenting on the first and last versions. Giulia Oskian, wise accomplice and a constant presence from afar – and for helpful observations on the second draft. Manos Tsakiris, humanist scientist, who knows what matters and makes transformative things happen, for his support, his inspiring research on interoception and the sense of self – and crucial comments on the final draft.

And: Alexandre Billon, for conversations on the self, philosophy and poetry over prolonged, noisy family meals. Laura Bossi, for her constant, affectionate support, and for sharing her wisdom and her immense erudition about neurology, its history, and much else. Fay Bound Alberti, for her generous support and bold work on the body in history. Pia Campeggiani, for her keen, enthusiastic reading of these pages and her clear thinking about emotions. Margherita Castellani, who has long understood it all, and for responding to this book as she did. Antonio Damasio, for his indispensable ideas and writings, for buoying exchanges, and for his all-round encouragement. Ophélia Deroy, for her provocative research, generosity, and free spirit. Maya Gratier, for our unending conversation, for her insights into infant development, and for helping me understand how I had to restructure the book. Deborah Levy, for her wisdom, and for telling me that another draft was needed. Helga Nowotny, for talks about science and more over happy meals in lovely places. Pasquale Pasquino, for reading and appreciating a raw first draft in Sicily, before anyone else had seen it. Victor Pitron, for generously sharing his insights into functional ailments from the psychiatric front. Philippe Rochat, for our rich exchanges about time, mind, life, for his comments on various drafts, and his encouraging me to write more freely about my mother. Didier Sicard, doctor, ethicist and family friend, for his thoughtful comments and deontological observations early on. Justin E. H. Smith, for his lively erudition and curiosity and for making the 'Three Souls' conference happen, out of which much has grown. Dan Sperber, for all that he has taught over the decades. Miranda Spieler, passionate historian, for crucially entreating me to witness for myself, and for first intuiting, even before I knew it, that I should write about my mother.

More friends old and new – writers, scholars, journalists, performers, artists, curators – who heard about this as the project developed over the years, took interest, and shared ideas, insights and experiences, or asked questions that provoked or goaded me on: Maryam d'Abo, Lisa Appignanesi, Winsome Brown, Joan Juliet Buck, Craig Burnett, Ian Buruma, Giovanna Carravieri, Giulia Carrozzini, Roberto Casati, Emanuele Coccia, Rana Dasgupta, Rachel Donadio, Pamela Druckerman, Jennifer Dworkin, Cécile Dutheil de la Rochère, Lisa Dwan, Monique El-Faizy, Giovanni Frazzetto, Janine di Giovanni, Anthony Gottlieb, Moira Grassi, Myriam Haikel, Elisa de Halleux, Charlotte Hellman, Fiammetta Horvat, Leela Jacinto, John Krinsky, Simon Kuper, Natasha Lehrer, Mark Lilla, Sara Lipton, Françoise Longy, George Makari, Livia Manera, Sabine Matheson, Spencer Matheson, Orlando Mostyn-Owen, Turi Munthe, Dominique Nabokov, Marie d'Origny, Susan Orlando, Keren Osman, Anaël Pigeat, Camilla Pietrabissa, Julie Polidoro, Emilie Prattico, Maël Renouard, Elizabeth Rubin, Catherine Rubin-Kermorgant, Logan Sandridge, Irene Santori, the sadly late Gaia Servadio, Kamila Shamsie, Laura Spinney, Aurélia Thierrée, Yuliya Tsaplina, Ananya Vajpeyi, Aline Vaudan, Patricia Wheatley.

◆

My sister Alba Arikha who, as a novelist, urged me to base each chapter on a case, for her moral support, and, with her husband Tom Smail, for their hospitality in London and for being real family. My nephew Ascanio Branca and my niece Arianna Branca, for their sensitivity and swift minds. I finished one draft at the Roman home of Nella and Gigi Simonetta, whose hands-on devotion to their grandsons has been a great support.

My beloved, now late mother, Anne Atik, for her amazing vitality and humour, and for all the extraordinary riches that she gave me, and that are here to stay. She lived and died a poet, and one of her utterances became the poetic title to the book. It is especially poignant that she cannot read this. My equally beloved father, Avigdor Arikha, lived and died a painter, but he also inculcated in me a love of science that informs these pages, and showed me how art and science can, and perhaps must be tightly enmeshed.

The writing of this book went in spurts and stages. It was a slow learning curve, and the path to it took a while: by the time I had finished, my sons Vigo and Amos were old enough to understand that their mother had written a new book – and one 'about the brain' too, which, I told them, could perhaps help us understand what had happened to their grandmother, whom they lost just after it was finished. It is enlightening, humbling, and immensely happy to witness and partake in their development. Their father Marcello Simonetta, while writing his own books at record speed, stood fast, through turbulence and calm, sometimes taking a peek, spurring me on. I owe him loving thanks for all the beauty that we have shared over the years.

Copyright Acknowledgements

Notes

Chapter 1: The Double Mirror

1. Consciousness is a major topic of philosophical and
   interdisciplinary investigation with an enormous literature, and
   is not itself the subject of this book. For a brief but reliable
   survey of how the concept has been studied and defined over
   centuries and disciplines, see the online entry by Robert Van
   Gulick, 'Consciousness', in *The Stanford Encyclopedia of
   Philosophy* (Spring 2018 edition), https://plato.stanford.edu/
   entries/consciousness/. The scientific investigation of
   consciousness has grown hugely over the past two decades,
   and some aspects of the biological study of consciousness (for
   instance by the research groups at the Sackler Centre for
   Consciousness Science, University of Sussex) do encompass
   the themes of this book. One major definition of
   consciousness amongst philosophers and mind scientists today
   is that it consists in our having 'phenomenal experience': there
   is a 'what it is like' to have an experience. And arguably, one
   major feature of phenomenal experience of consciousness is
   that it is subjective, and that it comes with self-consciousness,
   or self-awareness – that is, the awareness that I am the subject
   of my perceptions, sensations and thoughts. This self-
   awareness, in turn, has been classically tested with the
   so-called mirror test, first performed in 1970 by evolutionary
   psychologist Gordon Gallup, 'Chimpanzees: Self-recognition',
   Science, 167: 3914, 2 January 1970, pp. 86–7. The test is passed

when the subject is capable of noticing a mark made on their face. Humans typically pass the test at around eighteen months. There is a sliding scale of awareness, too. Animals such as great apes, dolphins, some elephants and some birds including magpies, are capable of passing this test as well, though the test is not a fool-proof guarantee and is open to interpretation. Recent experiments with mice are showing a sensitivity to mirror image, though its nature is not yet clear: see Takeshi Ishihara et al., 'Behavioural Changes in Mice after Getting Accustomed to the Mirror', *Hindawi Behavioural Neurology*, vol. 2020, https://doi.org/10.1155/2020/4071315. Intepretations of the mirror test in humans have changed over the past decade. For developmental psychologist Philippe Rochat, self-recognition emerges earlier, while the mirror test signals a sense of shame, of being seen by others, and therefore the dawning of a social sensibility: see in particular Philippe Rochat and Dan Zahavi 'The Uncanny Mirror: A Re-framing of Mirror Self-experience', *Consciousness and Cognition*, 20, 2011, pp. 204–13, and Rochat et al., 'Social Awareness and Early Self-recognition', *Consciousness and Cognition*, 21: 3, September 2012, pp. 1,491–7.

2. To some extent, Descartes borrowed the structure of this argument from Augustine and his related notion that 'if I am mistaken, I exist' ('si fallor, sum'), in *City of God*, Book XI, 26. For an analysis of this borrowing, and of the logical, theological and metaphysical overlaps and differences between the two arguments, see for instance Roger Ariew, *Descartes Among the Scholastics* (Leiden and London: Brill, 2011), pp. 297, 310–12; Stephen Menn, *Descartes and Augustine* (Cambridge and New York, NY: Cambridge University Press, 1998), pp. 3–11 and passim; Michael Ayers, 'Theories of Knowledge and Belief', in Dan Garber and Michael Ayers, eds, *The Cambridge History of Seventeenth-Century Philosophy*, vol. 2 (Cambridge and New York, NY: Cambridge University Press, 1998); Gareth B. Matthews, *Thoughts's Ego in Augustine and Descartes* (Ithaca, NY and London: Cornell University Press, 1992).

3. Metacognition can be defined as 'thinking about thinking', and involves the operation of metarepresentation. These processes continue to be investigated within the cognitive sciences. See Dan Sperber, ed., *Metarepresentation: A Multidisciplinary Perspective* (Oxford and New York, NY: Oxford University Press, 2000). See also Joëlle Proust, 'Metacognition and Metarepresentation: Is a Self-directed Theory of Mind a Precondition for Metacognition?', *Synthese*, 159, 2007, pp. 271–95. Research is also ongoing into the putative metacognitive capacities of mammals such as apes, dolphins and rats, as well as birds such as pigeons. Evidence is not conclusive, especially with regard to cognition of one's own cognitive state, as opposed to world-directed metacognition, as pointed out by Peter Carruthers in 'Meta-cognition in Animals: A Skeptical Look', *Mind & Language*, 23:1, February 2008, pp. 58–9.

4. Note that for Descartes, medicine was one of the three highest domains of knowledge. As he wrote in the Preface to his *Principles of Philosophy* (1644), 'all Philosophy is like a tree, of which Metaphysics is the root, Physics the trunk, and all the other sciences the branches that grow out of this trunk, which are reduced to three principles, namely, Medicine, Mechanics, and Ethics' (tr. John Veitch).

5. Descartes developed this view in his *Les Passions de l'âme* (Paris, 1649) and in his philosophical correspondence with Princess Elisabeth of Bohemia from 1643 until his death in 1650.

6. See for instance Roselyne Rey, 'Psyche, Soma, and the Vitalist Philosophy of Medicine', in John P. Wright and Paul Potter, eds., *Psyche and Soma: Physicians and Metaphysicians on the Mind–Body Problem from Antiquity to Enlightenment* (Oxford: Clarendon Press, 2000), pp. 255–65.

7. Margaret Cavendish, *Philosophical Letters* (1664), 1.11. Also quoted by Siri Hustvedt in 'The Delusions of Certainty', in Siri Hustvedt, *A Woman Looking at Men Looking at Women* (New York, NY: Simon & Schuster, 2016), p. 145. This essay

by Hustvedt is also published as a self-standing e-book (New York, NY: Simon & Schuster, 2017), as well as a single volume in France and Italy.

8. See my *Passions and Tempers: A History of the Humours* (New York, NY: Ecco, HarperCollins, 2007).

9. Ribot 'proposed that mental disease would act as the experimental arm of psychology': see George Makari, *Revolution in Mind: The Creation of Psychoanalysis* (New York, NY: Harper, 2008), p. 13.

10. Spanish neuroscientist Santiago Ramón y Cajal (1852–1934) brought to light the functioning of nervous cells in 1887, which resulted in the neuron theory that is considered today the foundation of neuroscience. In 1906, German neurologist Korbinian Brodmann (1868–1918) mapped the areas of the brain according to their neuronal organization, and brain areas are still identified with their numbered Brodmann areas.

11. This is by no means a universally accepted point, given that belief in an immortal soul of some sort is common to most religions. At the time of writing, the philosophical position of 'panpsychism' has regained popularity – the notion that the universe itself is imbued with consciousness – but it is not one I consider here. A collection of philosophical essays on this topic is Godehard Brüntrup and Ludwig Jaskolla, eds, *Panpsychism: Contemporary Perspectives* (Oxford and New York, NY: Oxford University Press, 2016).

12. Behaviourism was in part a reaction to the subjective psychology developed by Wilhelm Wundt. See for instance, in Joshua W. Clegg, ed., *Self-Observation on the Social Sciences* (New Brunswick, NJ and London: Transaction, 2013), the essays by Adrian C. Brock, 'The History of Introspection Revisited', pp. 25–38, and Alan Costall, 'Introspection and the Myth of Methodological Behaviorism', pp. 67–78.

13. These corners are those of computationalism and 'strong AI'. I believe that those cognitivists for whom affect or emotion are irrelevant to the study of mind are holding on to a fantastical, naïve view of human nature. For Siri Hustvedt, it is also a

fantasy of transcending the biological, 'wet' body: see her 'The Delusions of Certainty' in Hustvedt, *A Woman Looking at Men Looking at Women*, passim, especially pp. 281–94.

14. The question of generalizability is a philosophical one, which corresponds to the question of how the scientific method can account for subjective experience at all. For a good overview of the debate, see Wayne Wu, 'The Neuroscience of Consciousness', in Edward N. Zalta, ed., *The Stanford Encyclopedia of Philosophy* (Winter 2018), https://plato.stanford.edu/entries/consciousness-neuroscience/

15. There is a vast and growing philosophical literature around the notion of 'enactivism' and of '4E cognition' as embodied, embedded, extended, enacted. See for instance Giovanna Colombetti, *Feeling Body: Affective Science Meets the Enactive Mind* (Cambridge, MA and London: MIT Press, 2017); Ezequiel Di Paolo, Thomas Buhrmann, and Xabier Barandiaran, *Sensorimotor Life: An Enactive Proposal* (Oxford and New York, NY: Oxford University Press, 2017); Shaun Gallagher, *Enactivist Interventions: Rethinking the Mind* (Oxford and New York, NY: Oxford University Press, 2017); and many others.

16. There does however remain a 'hard problem', so-called by philosophers of mind, of how it is that the complexity of personal experience, the literally mind-boggling phenomenon of consciousness and selfhood, can be accounted for by physiological and cellular activity. In other words, the mind is not *the same* as the brain. The expression 'hard problem' was coined by philosopher David Chalmers in 1995, in his now classic paper 'Facing Up to the Problem of Consciousness', *Journal of Consciousness Studies* 2: 3 (1995), pp. 200–19. The brain is known as the most complex object in the universe, with its 86 billion neurons (135 billion if one includes the cerebellum) and hundreds of trillions of synaptic connections: it isn't surprising that it developed the capacity of self-knowledge. But the hard problem states that even if we could unravel the whole mechanism, we wouldn't be able to unravel the stuff of experience, its 'qualia', or what it *feels like* to see

red, for instance. Experience does remain irreducible to what we know about physiology, and our very capacity to contemplate ourselves does remain mysterious. But attention to the body and the world in which the brain is ensconced has, in my view, somewhat diminished the importance of the hard problem: the mind can now be seen as an outcome of the processes which engage the whole organism that is subserved by the brain.

17. See Mériam Korichi, 'Nous sommes confrontés à des manifestations psychiatriques inédites', AOC, [or Analyse opinion critique], 30 May 2020, https://aoc.media/entretien/2020/05/29/victor-pitron-nous-sommes-confrontes-a-des-manifestations-psychiatriques-inedites/ for her interview with psychiatrist Victor Pitron about his experience at the Pitié-Salpêtrière Hospital's psychiatry ER during the Covid-19 pandemic in 2020.

18. For a history and appraisal of this development, see my essay 'The Interoceptive Turn', *Aeon*, June 2019, https://aeon.co/essays/the-interoceptive-turn-is-maturing-as-a-rich-science-of-selfhood. Material from this article informs much of this book as well. The literature on this topic is vast and expanding. Most recently, see Manos Tsakiris and Helena De Preester, eds, *The Interoceptive Mind: From Homeostasis to Awareness* (Oxford and New York, NY: Oxford University Press, 2019); Frédérique de Vignemont and Adrian J. T. Alsmith, eds, *The Subject's Matter: Self-Consciousness and the Body* (Cambridge, MA and London: MIT Press, 2017); and Shaun Gallagher, ed., *The Oxford Handbook of The Self* (Oxford and New York, NY: Oxford University Press, 2011).

19. Antonio Damasio, *Descartes's Error: Emotion, Reason, and the Human Brain* (New York, NY: Putnam, 1994/London: Macmillan Picador, 1995). Damasio's influential work takes its cue in part from Spinoza's view of affect as an aspect of mind – one of his books is entitled *Looking for Spinoza: Joy, Sorrow, and the Feeling Brain* (New York, NY: Harcourt, 2003) – which has become resonant in contemporary scientific and

philosophical circles. Damasio also takes his cue from William James's scientific psychology, as given in his *Principles of Psychology* (New York, NY: Henry Holt, 1890) and in his 1884 article in *Mind*, vol. IX, issue 34, 1 April 1884, pp. 188–205, 'What is an Emotion?' Here James argued that emotions are the product of the body's autonomic response, only thereafter translated as behaviour and experienced as feelings, and that consciousness is a continuous stream of embodied experiences. The resurgence of James is central to the current turn to the study of affect and body.

20. See in this regard the groundbreaking article by Aikaterini Fotopoulou and Manos Tsakiris, 'Mentalizing Homeostasis: The Social Origins of Interoceptive Inference', *Neuropsychoanalysis*, 19: 1, 2017, pp. 3–28. See also Dimitris Bolis and Leonhard Schilbach, '"I Interact Therefore I Am": The Self as a Historical Product of Dialectical Attunement', *Topoi*, 13 June 2018.

21. The so-called 'exploration-exploitation trade-off' is a notion developed within decision theory to explore how we choose between the new unknown – potentially rewarding but also unsafe – and the known and safe. See for instance Oded Berger-Tal et al., 'The Exploration–Exploitation Dilemma: A Multidisciplinary Framework', *PLoS One*, 10: 3, April 2014.

22. Patients can serve the interests of scientists. Throughout the early history of neuroanatomy, neurophysiology and neuropsychology in the nineteenth century, clinical observations of patients in whom a vascular accident, say, had led to a visible deficiency started filling in the picture of how the brain worked. For instance, in 1861, French physician Paul Broca was able to identify a region in the frontal part of the brain's left hemisphere as being crucial for speech after a patient had had a stroke affecting that area, which rendered him unable to speak – aphasic – though he was able to comprehend what was said. It is now called Broca's area. Of course, scientists can also serve the interests of patients: neurology makes use of findings in neuroscience, cognitive psychology, genetics, molecular biology, epidemiology and so

on. But rarely is the science immediately applicable to the person in need.

23. Thanks to Vittorio Gallese for pointing to 'dimensional' versus 'categorical' accounts.

24. The distinction between normal and pathological as partaking of quantity or quality, as state or process, category or dimension, was famously examined by medically trained historian and philosopher of science Georges Canguilhem, *Le normal et le pathologique* (Paris: Presses Universitaires de France, 1966). See also Jacques Joubert, 'Le normal et le pathologique: Relire Canguilhem', *Revue des sciences religieuses*, 73: 4, 1999, pp. 497–518.

25. There is a philosophical tradition of using the first-person insights we garner when we examine our very awareness: it is known as phenomenology, which I put into practice in the following pages, without however discussing it. The French philosopher Maurice Merleau-Ponty (1908–61) remains one of its most celebrated exponents. He was a follower of Edmund Husserl (1859–1938), as was Erwin Straus (1891–1975), a German-born, American-based neurologist who used a phenomenological approach to understand the mind and psychiatry. Merleau-Ponty began to be cited within the philosophically informed mind sciences in the 1990s, most famously in Francisco Varela, Evan Thompson, and Eleanor Rosch, *The Embodied Mind: Cognitive Science and Human Experience* (Cambridge, MA and London: MIT Press, 1991). Varela (1946–2001) still exerts influence within the philosophically informed neurosciences and psychology today, and within the philosophical school of 'enactivism': see above, n. 15.

Chapter 2: The Old Campus

1. Michel Foucault gave a bold, interpretive history of this period in his *Histoire de la folie à l'âge classique* (Paris: Gallimard, 1972).

2. German physician Johann Christian Reil is credited with coining the term 'psychiatry', in 1808. See for instance Jeanne Mesmin d'Estienne, 'La Folie selon Esquirol. Observations médicales et conceptions de l'aliénisme à Charenton entre 1825 et 1840', *Revue d'histoire du XIXe siècle*, 40, 2010, pp. 95–112, http://journals.openedition.org/rh19/3994

3. Philippe Pinel, *Nosographie philosophique ou méthode de l'analyse appliquée à la médecine* (Paris, 1798). Pinel based aspects of his nosology on that of the English physician William Cullen — who coined the term 'neurosis'. See also my *Passions and Tempers*, pp. 255–6.

4. Esquirol was greatly influenced by Scottish physician Alexander Crichton (1763–1856), author of *An Inquiry into the Nature and Origins of Mental Derangement, Comprehending a Concise System of Physiology and Pathology of the Human Mind, and History of the Passions and Their Effects* (London, 1798). See Dora B. Weiner 'Mind and Body in the Clinic: Philippe Pinel, Alexander Crichton, Dominique Esquirol, and the Birth of Psychiatry' in G. S. Rousseau, ed., *The Languages of Psyche: Mind and Body in Enlightenment Thought* (Berkeley, CA: University of California Press, 1990), pp. 331–90.

5. Later Esquirol was instrumental in bringing about the 1838 law finally conferring a social status on the 'aliénés' and officializing their institutional care in France.

6. Reference books that tell the broader history of neuroscience, neurology and psychiatry include Edwin Clarke and L. S. Jacyna, *Nineteenth-Century Origins of Neuroscientific Concepts* (Berkeley and Los Angeles, CA, and London: University of California Press, 1987); Stanley Finger, *Origins of Neuroscience: A History of Explorations into Brain Function* (New York, NY: Oxford University Press, 1994); German Berrios and Roy Porter, eds, *A History of Clinical Psychiatry: The Origin & History of Psychiatric Disorders* (London and New Brunswick, NJ: Athlone Press, 1995).

7. Other important clinicians connected to the so-called

Salpêtrière school include Alfred Binet, Georges Gilles de la Tourette and Jules Cotard, amongst others.

8. See Christopher G. Goetz, 'Jean-Martin Charcot and the Anatomo-clinical Method of Neurology', *Handbook of Clinical Neurology*, 2010, 95, ch. 15, pp. 203–12.

9. These technologies were first developed for such use by pioneering neurologist Guillaume-Benjamin Duchenne whom Pinel thought of as his master. Duchenne studied and wrote a treatise on physiognomics which greatly influenced Darwin in his study of the expression of the emotions, *Mécanisme de la physionomie humaine, ou analyse électro-physiologique de l'expression des passions* (Paris: Jules Renouard, 1862).

10. See Santiago Giménez-Roldán, 'Clinical History of Blanche Wittman and Current Knowledge of Psychogenic Non-epileptic Seizures', *Neurosciences and History*, 4: 4, 2016, pp. 122–9, and Julien Bogousslavsky, 'Hysteria after Charcot: Back to the Future', in Julien Bogousslavsky, ed., *Following Charcot: A Forgotten History of Neurology and Psychiatry* (Basel: Karger, 2011): *Frontiers in Neurology and Neuroscience*, 29, pp. 137–61.

11. Both hysteria and hypochondria are, in nosological history, connected to melancholy, in particular as described by Robert Burton in his great magnum opus *The Anatomy of Melancholy*, first published in 1621. See for instance my 'As a Lute Out of Tune', *Public Domain Review*, 1 May 2013, https://publicdomainreview.org/essay/as-a-lute-out-of-tune-robert-burtons-melancholy

12. On the evolution of asylums, see Roy Porter, *Madness: A Brief History* (Oxford and New York, NY: Oxford University Press, 2002), pp. 89–122.

13. Pierre-Adolphe Piorri, *Clinique médicale de l'hôpital de la Pitié (Service de la Faculté de Médecine) et de l'Hospice de la Salpêtrière en 1832* (Paris and London: Baillière, 1833), pp. 264–76.

14. As George Makari writes in *Revolution in Mind*: 'Charcot had conquered hysteria and hypnotism by conceptualizing these mysteries as nothing more than inherited neural dysfunctions that resulted in altered states of consciousness' (p. 30).

15. Lisa Appignanesi, *Mad, Bad and Sad: A History of Women and the Mind Doctors from 1800 to the Present* (London: Virago, 2008), pp. 129–30. This is within her very insightful chapter on hysteria, Charcot and Freud, pp. 125–46.

16. A helpful account of Charcot's famous sessions and of the complexity of the historiography is Elaine Showalter's essay 'Hysteria, Feminism, and Gender', in Sander L. Gilmanet et al., *Hysteria Beyond Freud* (Berkeley, CA: University of California Press, 1993), pp. 286–336: 307–15. The book is an in-depth analysis of the notion of hysteria throughout its convoluted history. See also Christopher G. Goetz, 'Charcot and the Myth of Misogyny', *Neurology*, 52: 8, May 1999.

17. Freud broke off from clinical study once he realized that the neurological sciences of his day did not yet have the measure of yielding the secrets of the mind. His break from Charcot involved developing Bernheim's claim that suggestibility was the mechanism at work in hypnosis, and interpreting this mechanism as the unconscious 'autosuggestion' that became central to the psychoanalytic process: Makari, *Revolution in Mind*, pp. 33–7. He also distanced himself from Charcot's degeneration theory, in large part because it took Jewish families as an example. See also Jean Clair, ed., *Freud: du regard à l'écoute* (Paris: Gallimard/Musée d'art et d'histoire du Judaïsme, 2018).

18. Sigmund Freud and Joseph Breuer, *Studies in Hysteria* (first published as *Studien über Hysterie* (Vienna, 1895)), trans. Nicola Lockhurst (London and New York: Penguin, 2004), pp. 25–50: p. 34. The case of 'Fraülein Anna O.', the first in the book, was written by Breuer. Her real name was Bertha Pappenheim.

19. Emil Kraepelin (1856–1926), Aloïs Alzheimer (1864–1915). Kraepelin included the neurodegenerative disease that the latter discovered in his 1910 edition of his handbook on psychiatry: *Psychiatrie*, 8th edn, vol. 1: *Allgemeine Psychiatrie*; vol 2: *Klinische Psychiatrie* (Leipzig: Barth, 1909, 1910). See Hanns Hippius and Gabriele Neundörfer, 'The Discovery of

Alzheimer's Disease', *Dialogues in Clinical Neuroscience*, 5: 1, March 2003, pp. 101–8.

20. As the psychoanalyst John Bowlby wrote, 'The categorists are still searching for diagnostic criteria that distinguish the mentally ill from the normal, though today their search is more likely to be for genetically determined biochemical anomalies than for any behavioural criterion. [On the other hand, there are] those others who, like myself, believe continuity to be a more fruitful perspective.' This is cited in Georgina L. Barnes et al., 'John Bowlby and Contemporary Issues of Clinical Diagnosis', *Attachment*, 12: 1, August 2018, pp. 35–47.

21. See, most explicitly: Michael Fitzgerald, 'Do Psychiatry and Neurology Need a Close Partnership or a Merger?' *British Journal of Psychiatry Bulletin*, 39: 3, June 2015, pp. 105–7; Victor Pitron et al., 'Troubles somatiques fonctionnels: un modèle cognitif pour mieux les comprendre/Functional Somatic Syndromes: A Comprehensive Cognitive Model', *Société Nationale Française de Médecine Interne*, 2019, pp. 466–73; Vaughan Bell et al., 'What is the Functional/Organic Distinction Actually Doing in Psychiatry and Neurology?' version 1; peer review: 1 approved, *Wellcome Open Research*, 5: 138, 2020.

Chapter 3: The Lost Years

1. Plato, *Meno*: 'learning and inquiry are nothing but recollection' (81b–c). For an analysis of the concept, see the essay by philosopher and foremost Plato translator Reginald E. Allen, 'Anamnesis in Plato's *Meno* and *Phaedo*', *Review of Metaphysics*, 13: 1, September 1959, pp. 165–74.

2. A similar case of post-injury focal retrograde amnesia (FRA) is presented and analysed, along with the patient's neuropsychological data, in Pascale Piolino et al., 'Right Ventral Frontal Hypometabolism and Abnormal Sense of Self

in a Case of Disproportionate Retrograde Amnesia', *Cognitive Neuropsychology*, 22: 8, December 2005, pp. 1,005–34.

3. Cognitive neuroscientist Endel Tulving, known for his important research on memory, was the first to make this distinction, in 1985, in 'Memory and Consciousness' *Canadian Psychology/Psychologie canadienne*, 26(1), 1985, pp. 1–12: 'Speculations supported by empirical observations are offered concerning different memory systems (procedural, semantic, and episodic) and corresponding varieties of consciousness (anoetic, noetic, and autonoetic), with special emphasis on episodic memory and autonoetic consciousness as its necessary correlate. Evidence relevant to these speculations is derived from a case study of an amnesic patient who is conscious in some ways but not in others, as well as from simple experiments on recall and recognition by normal subjects. Autonoetic (self-knowing) consciousness is the name given to the kind of consciousness that mediates an individual's awareness of his or her existence and identity in subjective time extending from the personal past through the present to the personal future. It provides the characteristic phenomenal flavour of the experience of remembering' (p. 1). See also the more recent Marie P. Vanderkeckhove, 'Memory, Autonoetic Consciousness and the Self: Consciousness as a Continuum of Stages', *Self and Identity*, 8: 1, 2009, pp. 4–23; Janet Metcalfe and Lisa K. Son, 'Anoetic, Noetic and Autonoetic Metacognition', in Michael J. Beran et al., eds, *Foundations of Metacognition* (Oxford and New York, NY: Oxford University Press, 2012), pp. 289–301. And see Siri Hustvedt, 'Pace, Space and the Other in the Making of Fiction', *Costellazioni*: 5, 2018, pp. 23–50: as she writes, reflective self-consciousness 'is the ability to reflect upon, represent, and narrate one's own thoughts, actions, and life as a whole. This appears to require a particular kind of explicit, declarative memory, also called autobiographical memory, noetic, or extended consciousness, an ability to turn oneself into an other to oneself in memory and fantasy' (p. 31).

4. See Robin G. Morris and Daniel C. Mograbi, 'Anosognosia,

Autobiographical Memory and Self-knowledge in Alzheimer's Disease', *Cortex*, 49, 2013, pp. 1,553–65, 'episodic memory also contributes to a sense of self, allowing autonoetic consciousness, time and travel and re-experiencing of details' (p. 1,554).

5. Neuroscientist Martin A. Conway, who researches memory, has developed a 'Self-Memory System (SMS)', which, as he outlines in the abstract of 'Memory and the Self', *Journal of Memory and Language*, 53 (2005), pp. 594–628, 'is a conceptual framework that emphasizes the interconnectedness of self and memory. Within this framework memory is viewed as the data base of the self. The self is conceived as a complex set of active goals and associated self-images, collectively referred to as the *working self.* The relationship between the working self and long-term memory is a reciprocal one in which autobiographical knowledge constrains what the self is, has been, and can be, whereas the working self modulates access to long-term knowledge' (p. 594). As he writes further: 'it has often been observed and long been known that memories may be altered, distorted, even fabricated, to support current aspects of the self' (p. 599). And as noted by Morris and Mograbi, 'Anosognosia, Autobiographical Memory and Self Knowledge in Alzheimer's Disease' (2013), Conway's notion of a 'working self' 'modulates encoding of new information based on goals and self-image. Here, memory provides continuity to the experience of selfhood by allowing storage of past information and the ability to project future scenarios (Addis and Tippett, 2004)' (p. 1,554). For an earlier, insightful account of the centrality of memory to the embodied sense of self and consciousness, see Israel Rosenfield, *The Strange, Familiar, and Forgotten: An Anatomy of Consciousness* (New York, NY: Vintage, 1993).

6. Théodule Ribot (1839–1916), *Les maladies de la mémoire* (Paris: Baillière, 1881), pp. 94–5.

7. Daniel L. Schacter, *Searching for Memory: The Brain, the Mind, and the Past* (New York, NY: Basic Books, 1996), p. 84.

8. See for instance Aimée M. Surprenant and Ian Neath, *Principles of Memory: Essays in Cognitive Psychology* (Hove, E. Sussex, and New York, NY: Psychology Press, 2009), p. 150.

9. See n. 5 above, and the observation by Martin Conway that 'memories may be altered, distorted, even fabricated, to support current aspects of the self'. Vanessa's 'working self' may have been effectively modulating her 'access to long-term knowledge' – too effectively. But even then, how and why did this occur after her coma?

10. Morris and Mograbi, 'Anosognosia, Autobiographical Memory and Self Knowledge in Alzheimer's Disease' (2013) write of 'the need to keep coherence between a sense of self and memories', which may explain why one will tend to have better recall of positive rather than negative memories. In their words, 'memory, especially autobiographical memory, is constrained to be coherent with an individual's goals, self-beliefs and self-representations (Conway 2005); this is in agreement with research which suggests the influence of self-reference or previous knowledge on encoding, consolidation and retrieval of new memories' (p. 1558).

11. Throughout history, memory has tended to be compared to whatever recording technology was current at the time. For an account of this, see Douwe Draaisma, *Metaphors of Memory: A History of Ideas about the Mind* (Cambridge: Cambridge University Press, 2000).

12. The name 'Transient Global Amnesia' was coined in two papers published in 1958 and 1964, by two neurologists at Boston's Massachusetts General Hospital, C. Miller Fisher and Raymond Adams: C. M. Fisher and R. D. Adams, 'Transient Global Amnesia', *Transactions of the American Neurological Association*, 83, 1958, pp. 143–6, and 'Transient Global Amnesia', *Acta Neurologica Scandinavica* 40, supp. 9, 1964, pp. 1–83. Fisher, a specialist of stroke, was a mentor for many neurologists.

13. See Steven Shapin, 'The Man who Forgot Everything', *New Yorker*, 14 October 2013, and the account by the scientist who

studied Molaison for decades: Suzanne Corkin, *Permanent Present Tense: The Unforgettable Life of the Amnesic Patient, H. M.* (New York, NY: Basic Books, 2013). See also Antonio Damasio, *The Feeling of What Happens: Body, Emotion and the Making of Consciousness* (New York, NY: Harcourt, 1999/ London: William Heinemann, 2000), pp. 113–21, where Damasio tells of a patient of his, David, who, following a viral encephalitis that damaged his hippocampus, was like HM unable to form new memories, but was also unable to recall old facts because of additional damage to other areas in the temporal lobe, in particular the inferotemporal and polar cortices. The loss is even more devastating than in the case of HM. His 'core consciousness' remains (p. 117), but 'his autobiographical memory has been reduced to a skeleton, and thus the autobiographical self that can be constructed at any moment is severely impoverished' (p. 119).

14. For an insightful account of this film, see Nathan Senn, 'Cultivating Self in the Other in Hirokazu Kore-eda's *Without Memory* (1996)', *Senses of Cinema*, June 2017, http://sensesofcinema.com/2017/cteq/without-memory/

15. Sergei Korsakoff was a nineteenth-century Russian psychiatrist who developed this very syndrome after years of alcoholism.

16. See Stanley B. Klein and Shaun Nichols, 'Memory and the Sense of Personal Identity', *Mind*, 121: 483, July 2012, pp. 677–702.

17. The notion of a core self has a wide literature, and was developed in depth by Antonio Damasio in *Self Comes to Mind: Constructing the Conscious Brain* (New York, NY: Random House/London: William Heinemann, 2010). The notion is tied into that of the levels and types of selfhood. William James wrote a key discussion about it in the chapter 'The Consciousness of Self' in his *The Principles of Psychology* (1890) (Cambridge, MA and London: Harvard University Press, 1981), pp. 279–379, vol. 1 ch. 10, developing the notion of a 'spiritual self' as distinct from 'the material self' and 'the social self', as well as from 'the pure Ego'. Philosopher Dan Zahavi studies the phenomenology of selfhood, and has argued for a 'minimal

self': see for instance his *Subjectivity and Selfhood: Investigating the First-Person Perspective* (Cambridge, MA: MIT Press, 2006). Philosopher Shaun Gallagher has been investigating the embodied sense of self: see for instance his *How the Body Shapes the Mind* (Oxford: Oxford University Press, 2005).

18. See David R. Euston, Aaron J. Gruber, and Bruce L. McNaughton, 'The Role of Medial Prefrontal Cortex in Memory and Decision Making', *Neuron*, 76: 6, 20 December 2012, pp. 1,057–70. See also Damasio, *Descartes's Error*, p. 134.

19. A similar case of 'focal retrograde amnesia', or FRA, is analysed by Pascale Piolino et al., 'Right Ventral Frontal Hypometabolism and Abnormal Sense of Self in a Case of Disproportionate Retrograde Amnesia', *Cognitive Neuropsychology*, 22, 2005, pp. 1–30.

20. A. R. Luria, *The Mind of a Mnemonist: A Little Book about a Vast Memory* (Cambridge, MA and London: Harvard University Press, 1968).

21. Reed Johnson, 'The Mystery of S., the Man with an Impossible Memory', *New Yorker*, 12 August 2017.

22. See Onno van der Hart and Rutger Horst, 'The Dissociation Theory of Pierre Janet', *Journal of Traumatic Stress*, 2: 4, 1989. See also Quinton Deeley, 'Hypnosis as a Model of Functional Neurologic Disorders', *Handbook of Clinical Neurology*, 139, 2016, pp. 95–103, where he writes: 'suggestion mediated the effects of ideas on hysteric symptoms through as yet unknown effects on brain activity'. Deeley offers an in-depth review of studies of functional symptoms, including hysterical paralysis, which used neuroimaging techniques. He refers in particular to a set of experiments by Yann Cojan et al., 'Motor Inhibition in Hysterical Conversion Paralysis', *NeuroImage* 47, 2009, pp. 1,026–37, which suggest that 'conversion symptoms do not act through cognitive inhibitory circuits, but involve selective activations in midline brain regions associated with self-related representations and emotion regulation.' In both functional paralysis and hypnosis, writes Deeley, Cojan's team 'reported increased functional connectivity between the motor cortex

and precuneus, proposing that in both cases motor inhibition (paralysis) may be mediated through mental imagery and self-reflective processing rather than executive inhibition.'

23. Makari, *Revolution in Mind*, pp. 31–2.

24. James, *The Principles of Psychology*, vol. 1, ch. 10, pp. 363–9.

25. Psychiatrist Allen J. Frances, who headed the committee for the elaboration of *DSM 4*, has been a severe critic of *DSM 5*. On the introduction in that edition of the appellation of SSD, see his blog post 'Mislabeling Medical Illness as Mental Disorder: The Eleventh *DSM 5* Mistake Needs an Eleventh Hour Correction', *Psychology Today*, 8 December 2012, https://www.psychologytoday.com/gb/blog/dsm5-in-distress/201212/mislabeling-medical-illness-mental-disorder

26. See Siri Hustvedt, 'I Wept for Four Years and When I Stopped I Was Blind', *Neurophysiologie Clinique/Clinical Neurophysiology*, 44: 4, October 2014, pp. 305–13, reprinted in Hustvedt, *A Woman Looking at Men*: 'Janet theorized a split of consciousness or dissociation in hysteria, which he posited as a psychobiological phenomenon that caused a pathological "retraction of consciousness," and he specifically related this retraction to the problem of agency' (p. 404).

27. Oliver Sacks, 'Speak, Memory', *New York Review of Books*, 21 February 2013.

28. See for instance, Sam McKenzie and Howard Eichenbaum, 'Consolidation and Reconsolidation: Two Lives of Memories?', *Neuron* 71: 2, 28 July 2011, pp. 224–33; Daniela Schiller and Elizabeth A. Phelps, 'Does Reconsolidation Occur in Humans?', *Frontiers in Behavioral Neuroscience*, May 2011, vol. 5: 24.

29. Yadin Dudai, Avi Karni, and Jan Born, 'The Consolidation and Transformation of Memory', *Neuron* 88: 1, 7 October 2015, pp. 20–32.

30. See also Siri Hustvedt, *The Shaking Woman or A History of My Nerves* (New York, NY: Picador, 2009), p. 108.

31. Vladimir Nabokov, *Speak, Memory* (London: Gollancz, 1951). Nabokov revised the text, and re-issued it in 1966 as *Speak, Memory: An Autobiography Revisited* (New York, NY: Vintage),

and wrote in the foreword: 'I revised many passages and tried to do something about the amnesic effects of the original – blank spots, blurry areas, domains of dimness' (p. 9).

32. Saint Augustine, trans. R. S. Pine-Coffin, *Confessions*, Book XI (London and New York, NY: Penguin, 1961), pp. 253–80.

33. Siri Hustvedt writes in *The Shaking Woman*: 'The faculty of memory cannot be separated from the imagination. They go hand in hand. To one degree or another, we all invent our personal pasts. And for most of us those pasts are built from emotionally colored memories. Affects give meaning to experience as *value*, as some philosophers put it. What we don't care about we forget' (p. 112).

34. Aquinas took his cue in particular from Aristotle. See for instance Anthony J. Lisska, *Aquinas's Theory of Perception: An Analytic Reconstruction*: 'The Imagination and Phantasia' (Oxford and New York, NY: Oxford University Press, 2016).

35. Paul Schilder was a forerunner of the study of disorders in body image: see his *The Image and Appearance of the Human Body* (New York, NY: International University Presses, 1950). Over the past two decades, research in this area has multiplied enormously, especially regarding the relation between body ownership and interoceptive processes. See for instance, Aikaterini Fotopoulou et al., 'Sense of Body Ownership in Patients Affected by Functional Motor Symptoms (Conversion Disorder)', *Consciousness and Cognition* 39, January 2016, pp. 70–76; Deborah Badoud and Manos Tsakiris, 'From the Body's Viscera to the Body's Image: Is There a Link Between Interoception and Body Image Concerns?' *Neuroscience and Biobehavioral Reviews*, 77, June 2017, pp. 237–46.

36. See for instance, Sinéad L. Mullall and Eleanor A. Maguire, 'Memory, Imagination, and Predicting the Future: A Common Brain Mechanism?' *The Neuroscientist*, 2014, 20: 3, pp. 220–34.

37. Hustvedt, 'I Wept for Four Years' (2014), p. 405.

38. Thanks to Katerina Fotopoulou and Siri Hustvedt for a conversation on this topic, and to Siri Hustvedt for her crucial comments on a previous version of this chapter, all of which

helped me rethink this case. See Siri Hustvedt, 'Philosophy Matters in Brain Matters', *Seizure* 22, 2013, pp. 169–73, where she writes: 'Every phenomenal thought and feeling is accompanied by brain changes' (p. 170), referring to Stanley Cobb, *Borderlands of Psychiatry* (Cambridge, MA: Harvard University Press, 1943): 'Anyone who stops to think realizes that no function is possible without an organ that is functioning and therefore no function takes place without structural change' (pp. 19–20).

39. Putative neurological functions are emerging for retrograde amnesia involving the loss of autonoetic memory. See for instance Hirokazu Kikuchi, 'Neural Basis of Dissociative Amnesia', *Higher Brain Function Research*, 31: 3, 2011, pp. 319–27: 'Studies with functional neuroimaging techniques have revealed functional abnormality of dissociative amnesia at brain level. There are two theories about brain mechanisms of dissociative amnesia: frontal executive inhibition of the medial temporal memory system, and functional disconnection of right fronto-temporal regions engaged in triggering autobiographical memory retrieval. Recent studies have reported evidence supporting each of the two theories' (abstract). See also Victor I. Reus, 'Psychogenic Amnesia and Fugue', in *Aminoff's Neurology and General Medicine*, 5th edition (2014), ch. 52, 'Functional Neurologic Symptom Disorders'. Reus writes: 'Although evidence of structural neurologic damage is, by definition, absent, recent research involving functional neuroimaging has identified state-dependent decreases in prefrontal cortex and right temporal frontal metabolism in patients with psychogenic amnesia that normalized with memory recovery following psychologic treatment. Hypometabolism in the insula, which seems involved in the ability to project oneself in time, has also been observed in patients with psychogenic amnesia. Such data may serve to support the conceptualization of psychogenic amnesia as a brain-based "disconnection syndrome" and facilitate therapeutic interventions that are humane and psychologically supportive in nature.'

40. See n. 22 above and Quinton Deeley's review of possible avenues for further neurological investigation of functional syndromes.
41. See Morris and Mograbi, 'Anosognosia, Autobiographical Memory and Self Knowledge in Alzheimer's Disease' (2013), pp. 1,553–65.

Chapter 4: Haunted

1. Théodule Ribot, *La Psychologie des sentiments* (Paris: Félix Alcan, 1896), p. 54.
2. The possible neurological aetiology of a similar case is described by Baland Jalal and Vilayanur S. Ramachandran in 'Sleep Paralysis, "The Ghostly Bedroom Intruder"' and 'Out-of-Body Experiences: The Role of Mirror Neurons', *Frontiers in Human Neuroscience*, February 2017, vol. 11:92, and by Mariateresa Sestito et al., in 'Embodying the Self: Neurophysiological Perspectives on the Psychopathology of Anomalous Bodily Experiences', *Frontiers in Human Neuroscience*, February 2017, vol. 11: 631.
3. Oliver Sacks, *Hallucinations* (New York, NY: Knopf, 2012).
4. Jean-Baptiste Esquirol, *Des Maladies mentales considérées sous le rapport médical, hygiénique et médico-légal* (Paris: J. B. Baillière, 1838, 2 vols): 'Un homme qui a la conviction intime d'une sensation actuellement perçue, alors que nul objet extérieur propre à exciter cette sensation n'est à la portée de ses sens, est dans un état hallucinatoire: c'est un visionnaire' (vol. 1, p. 188).
5. See Renaud Jardri et al., 'Cortical Activations During Auditory Verbal Hallucinations in Schizophrenia: A Coordinate-based Meta-analysis', *American Journal of Psychiatry*, 168: 1, January 2011, pp. 73–81.
6. Ibid., p. 159. See also Rafael Huertas, 'Between Doctrine and Clinical Practice: Nosography and Semiology in the Work of Jean-Etienne-Dominique Esquirol (1772–1840)', *History of Psychiatry*, 19: 2, pp. 123–40: pp. 131–3; also Guy Gimenez, Magali Guimont, and Jean-Louis Pedinielli, 'Etude de

l'évolution du concept d'hallucination dans la littérature psychiatrique classique', *L'Evolution psychiatrique*, 68: 2, 2003, pp. 289–98.

7. See David Baumeister et al., 'Auditory Verbal Hallucinations and Continuum Models of Psychosis: A Systematic Review of the Healthy Voice-Hearer Literature', *Clinical Psychology Review*, 51, 2017, pp. 125–41.

8. Sacks, *Hallucinations*, p. 237.

9. See Albert R. Powers et al., 'Paracingulate Sulcus Length is Shorter in Voice-Hearers Regardless of Need for Care', *Schizophrenia Bulletin*, 20 May 2020.

10. Ibid., p. 64.

11. See G. Lynn Stephens and George Graham, *When Self-consciousness Breaks: Alien Voices and Inserted Thoughts* (Cambridge, MA and London: MIT Press, 2000), p. 103, cited in Gottfried Vosgerau and Albert Newen, 'Thoughts, Motor Actions, and the Self', *Mind and Language*, 22: 1, February 2007, pp. 22–43: 'many people who experience voices are not having auditory hallucinations. They do not mistake their awareness of inner speech for auditory perception of somebody else's speech, nor do they even have the impression that they are hearing another speak. Thus, verbal hallucinations cannot be regarded, in general, as an audition-like experience' (p. 38).

12. The term 'vesania', and Pinel's nosology of 1798, derived from the influential nosology of Scottish physician William Cullen, which had appeared in Latin in 1769 as *Synopsis Nosologiae Methodicae*. The English translation of William Creech was published in 1800 as *Nosology: or, a Systematic arrangement of diseases, by classes, orders, genera, and species; with the distinguishing characters of each, and outlines of the systems of Sauvages, Linnæus, Vogel, Sagar, and Macbride* (Edinburgh: C. Stewart, 1800).

13. Originally from Greek, melancholy signified 'black bile', one of the four humours that for so long were believed to constitute the human organism. See my *Passions and Tempers*.

14. Philippe Pinel, *Traité médico-philosophique sur l'aliénation mentale*

(Paris: J. A. Brosson, 1809). For Pinel, diseases were fixed entities, organic disruptions that were categorizable in much the same way that plants were. He constructed his nosology in the lineage of the Enlightenment classifications of natural kinds, and on the basis of the *Nosologia methodica*, published in 1763, of physicist and botanist François Boissier de Sauvages, who was himself influenced by the great Swedish naturalist and botanist Carl von Linné. See Marc-Antoine Crocq, 'French Perspectives on Psychiatric Classification', *Dialogues in Clinical Neuroscience*, 17: 1, 2015, pp. 51–72, for a description of Sauvages's classification: 'Mental disorders, *Vesaniae*, belonged to the 8th class of diseases, which comprised four orders: (i) *Hallucinations*, subdivided into Vertigo, Suffusion, Diplopia, Syrigmus (ie, imaginary noise perceived in the ear), Hypochondriasis, and Somnambulism; (ii) *Morositates*, further subdivided into Pica, Bulimia, Polydipsia, Antipathia, Nostalgia, Panophobia (ie, panic terror), Satyriasis, Nymphomania, Tarantism (ie, immoderate craving for dance), and Hydrophobia; (iii) *Deliria*, subdivided into Paraphrosine (ie, temporary delirium caused by a substance or a medical illness), Amentia ('universal' delirium without furor), Melancholia ('partial' and nonaggressive delirium with sadness and chronicity), Mania ('universal delirium' with furor and chronicity), Demonomania (ie, melancholia attributed to the devil); and (iv) Folies anomales comprising Amnesia, and Agrypnia (ie, insomnia)' (p. 52).

15. Esquirol's definition, from his *Des Maladies Mentales Considérées Sous Les Rapports Médical, Hygiénique Et Médico-légal*, vol. 1 (1838), ch. 8 : 'De la Lypémanie ou Mélancolie', p. 200, is quoted in Paul Lefebvre 'Le traité des maladies mentales d'Esquirol: cent cinquante ans après', *Histoire des Sciences Médicales*, vol. 25: 2, 1991, pp. 169–74: 'La monomanie est caractérisée par une passion gaie ou triste, excitante ou oppressive, produisant le délire fixe et permanent, des désirs et des déterminations relatifs au caractère de la passion dominante, se divise naturellement en monomanie proprement

dite, ayant pour signe caractéristique un délire partiel et une passion excitante ou gaie, et en monomanie caractérisée par un délire partiel et une passion triste et oppressive . . . Je lui consacre le nom de monomanie . . . La seconde correspond à la mélancolie des anciens . . . à la mélancolie avec délire de Pinel. Malgré la crainte d'être accusé de néologisme, je lui donne le nom de lypémanie' (p. 170).

16. A history of the clinical notion of delusion is in Berrios and Porter, eds, *A History of Clinical Psychiatry*: ch. 14, 'Delusional Disorder'; 'Clinical Section', by Kenneth S. Kendler, pp. 360–171, and ch. 15, 'Social Section', by I. Dowbiggin, pp. 372–83.

17. Sir Thomas Browne, *Pseudodoxia Epidemica, Or, Enquiries, Into Very many received Tenents And commonly presumed Truths* (London, 1646), ch. 18: 'Of Moles, or Molls'. He writes 'For if vision be abolished, it is called *cæcitas*, or blindness; if depraved and receive its objects erroneously, Hallucination.'

18. See Bodil Kråkvik et al., 'Prevalence of Auditory Verbal Hallucinations in a General Population: A Group Comparison Study', *Scandinavian Journal of Psychology*, 56: 5, October 2015, pp. 508–15.

19. For decades, there prevailed the assumption that dreams occured mostly in the phase of so-called REM or paradoxical sleep, when, while the body is at its most immobilized and least receptive to external inputs, the brain is highly active, producing our sensorially rich dreams. Since then it has been shown that oneiric events, although they are highly concentrated during REM sleep, can occur at any time during the sleep cycle, including as one falls into and out of sleep. See for instance Mark Solms and Oliver Turnbull, *The Brain and the Inner World: An Introduction to the Neuroscience of Subjective Experience* (London: Karnac, 2002), pp. 182–96.

20. Suzanne K. Langer, *Philosophy in a New Key: A Study in the Symbolism of Reason, Rite, and Art* (Cambridge, MA: Harvard University Press, 1948/Toronto: Mentor, 1942), p. 46. See also the rich work on dreams and sleep of psychiatrist J. Allan

Hobson in 'REM Sleep and Dreaming: Towards a Theory of Protoconsciousness', *Nature Reviews Neuroscience*, 10 November 2009, pp. 803–14, where he advances the idea that dreams provide 'a virtual reality model of the world that is of functional use to the development and maintenance of waking consciousness' (abstract). He writes: 'dreaming is an indispensable . . . if sometimes misleading . . . subjective informant about what the brain does during REM sleep. Indeed, we may be bound to admit that dreaming itself could be an epiphenomenon without any direct effect on normal or abnormal cognition' (p. 805). See also Hustvedt, *The Shaking Woman*, pp. 128–39.

21. This was pointed out by pioneering sleep researcher Michel Jouvet in his *Le Sommeil et le rêve* (Paris: Odile Jacob, 1992), p. 132.

22. Esquirol, *Des Maladies mentales*, vol. 1 (1838), 'Des Hallucinations', pp. 192–3: 'Chez celui qui rêve, les idées de la veille se continuent pendant le sommeil; tandis que celui qui est en délire achève son rêve après qu'il est éveillé. Les rêves, comme les hallucinations, reproduisent toujours des idées anciennes.' And he continues: 'Comme dans le rêve, la série des images et des idées est quelquefois régulière, plus souvent les images et les idées se reproduisent dans le plus grand désordre, et offrent les associations les plus étranges. Comme dans le rêve, ceux qui ont des hallucinations ont quelquefois la conscience qu'ils sont dans le délire ou qu'ils rêvent, sans pouvoir dégager leur esprit. Celui qui rêve, celui qui a des hallucinations, n'est jamais étonné ni surpris des idées, des images qui le préoccupent, tandis qu'elles eussent excité tout son étonnement, s'il eut été éveillé ou s'il n'eût pas déliré. Ce phénomène, dans les deux circonstances, est causé par l'absence de toute idée accessoire, de toute image, avec laquelle celui qui rêve ou celui qui est halluciné puisse comparer l'objet de son rêve ou de son délire.'

23. See Jon S. Simons et al., 'The Neural Mechanisms of Hallucinations: A Quantitative Meta-analysis of Neuroimaging

Studies', *Neuroscience and Biobehavioral Reviews* 69, 2016, 113–23: 'dysfunctional activation in regions typically associated with episodic memory retrieval and with reality- and self-monitoring may facilitate the generation of erroneous percepts evoked via interactions between past memories and abnormal activity in sensory brain areas' (p. 123).

24. See Georg Northoff, *Neuro-Philosophy and the Healthy Mind: Learning from the Unwell Brain* (New York, NY and London: W. W. Norton, 2016): even when schizophrenics, he notes, 'do not hear a voice in the external environment, their auditory cortical resting-state activity is abnormally high. This is especially the case when they hear an internal voice, an auditory hallucination. Most interesting, when exposed to an external sound, these patients can no longer down-modulate their abnormally increased resting-state activity in the auditory cortex' (p. 157).

25. Sacks, *Hallucinations*, p. 237.

26. Victor Pitron and Frédérique de Vignemont, 'Beyond Differences Between the Body Schema and the Body Image: Insights from Body Hallucinations', *Consciousness and Cognition*, 53, 2017, pp. 115–21: 'The phenomenology of hallucinations resembles the phenomenology of perception so that one may be unaware that one is hallucinating' (p. 117).

27. Damasio, *Self Comes to Mind*, p. 20.

28. Damasio develops this in *The Strange Order of Things: Life, Feeling, and the Making of Cultures* (New York, NY: Random House, 2018), and, focusing on consciousness, in *Feeling and Knowing: Making Minds Conscious* (New York, NY: Pantheon, 2021).

29. Allostasis can be defined as 'the regulation of bodily states through change': see Anil K. Seth and Manos Tsakiris, 'Being a Beast Machine: The Somatic Basis of Selfhood', *Trends in Cognitive Sciences*, 22: 11, 1 November 2018, pp. 969–81: p. 972. See also Andrew W. Corcoran and Jakob Hohwy, 'Allostasis, Interoception, and the Free Energy Principle: Feeling Our Way Forward', in Tsakiris and de Preester, eds, *The Interoceptive Mind*, pp. 272–92. And see my, 'The Interoceptive Turn' (2019).

30. Karl Friston, 'The Mathematics of Mind-time', *Aeon*, 18 May 2017, https://aeon.co/amp/essays/consciousness-is-not-a-thing-but-a-process-of-inference. For a profile of Andy Clark and of his relation to Friston, see Larissa MacFarquhar, 'The Mind-Expanding Ideas of Andy Clark', *New Yorker*, 2 April 2018.

31. An accessible and reliable summary of this theory is in a profile of Karl Friston by Shaun Raviv, 'The Genius Neuroscientist Who Might Hold the Key to True AI', *Wired*, 13 November 2018. Thousands of scientific papers now make use of, implement, develop and also critique various aspects and implications of the theory of predictive processing.

32. Karl Friston, 'The Free-Energy Principle: A Unified Brain Theory?' *Nature Reviews Neuroscience*, 11, February 2010, pp. 127–38.

33. Roy Salomon et al., 'The Boundaries of the Self: The Sense of Agency Across Different Sensorimotor Aspects', *Journal of Vision*, 19(4): 14, 2019, pp. 1–11.

34. Anil K. Seth and Karl J. Friston, 'Active Interoceptive Inference and the Emotional Brain', *Philosophical Transactions of the Royal Society B*, 371: 1708, November 2016.

35. In David Benrimoh et al., 'Active Inference and Auditory Hallucinations', *Computational Psychiatry*, December 2018: 2, pp. 183–204, AVH are analysed in computational terms, as a case of 'false (positive) inference. Active inference treats perception as a process of hypothesis testing, in which sensory data are used to disambiguate between alternative hypotheses about the world. Crucially, this depends upon a delicate balance between prior beliefs about unobserved (hidden) variables and the sensations they cause. A false inference that a voice is present, even in the absence of auditory sensations, suggests that prior beliefs dominate perceptual inference' (abstract).

36. Philip R. Corlett et al., 'The Predictive Coding Account of Psychosis', *Biological Psychiatry*, 84, 1 November 2018, abstract and pp. 634–43. See also https://youtu.be/93vqcBLWK-8 and the field of computational psychiatry generally, notably the work of Chrstoph Mathys on hallucinations and delusions.

37. See Iris E. Sommer et al., 'Dissecting Auditory Verbal Hallucinations into Two Components: Audibility (Gedankenlautwerden) and Alienation (Thought Insertion)', *Psychopathology* 43: 2, February 2010, pp. 137–40. This is an account of AVH as instances of 'audibility', which results from 'a disinhibition of the auditory cortex in response to self-generated speech', as well as 'alienation' – inner speech is produced in the right hemisphere in AVH, rather than the left, which would explain why it is not experienced as self-generated, and therefore feels like 'thought insertion'.

38. For an in-depth account of how the Bayesian model can account for AVH, see Clara S. Humpton et al., 'From Computation to the First-Person: Auditory-verbal Hallucinations and Delusions of Thought Interference in Schizophrenia-spectrum Psychoses', *Schizophrenia Bulletin*, 45, supp. 1, pp. S56–66, 2019, a review article bridging computational and phenomenological approaches: 'The "comparator" or "inner speech model" is an influential model of AVH based on predictive motor processes . . . It proposes that efference copies of motor commands are sent to a "forward model" that uses them to predict their sensory consequences in advance of sensory feedback. Successful prediction may attenuate the perception of those sensory consequences and also result in the feeling of agency for a movement, whereas prediction errors may lead one to infer the environment or some other agent was responsible for the discrepancy . . . In AVH, the sensation that AVH come from someone else/another source other than one's self could also be accounted for by failures in self-monitoring' (p. S59).

39. See Tim Shallice and Francesca Borgo, 'Category Specificity and Feature Knowledge: Evidence from New Sensory-Quality Categories', *Cognitive Neuropsychology*, 20: 3/4/5/6, 2003, pp. 327–53.

40. A very similar case is reported by Yves Agid et al. in 'Hallucinations, REM Sleep, and Parkinson's Disease: A Medical Hypothesis', *Medical Hypothesis*, 55: 2, 25 July 2000.

41. Damasio, *The Strange Order of Things*, p. 51.
42. Guillermo Horga et al., 'A Perceptual Inference Mechanism for Hallucinations Linked to Striatal Dopamine', *Current Biology* 28, 19 February 2018, pp. 503–14: 'These findings outline a novel dopamine-dependent mechanism for perceptual modulation in physiological conditions and further suggest that this mechanism may confer vulnerability to hallucinations in hyper-dopaminergic states underlying psychosis' (abstract). See also Anil K. Seth, Keisuke Suzuki, and Hugo D. Critchley, 'An Interoceptive Predictive Coding Model of Conscious Presence', *Frontiers in Psychology*, 10 January 2012.
43. See David Sulzer et al., 'Striatal Dopamine Neurotransmission: Regulation of Release and Uptake', *Basal Ganglia*, 6: 3, August 2016, pp. 123–48.
44. A DaTscan is used in particular for Parkinson's diagnoses. It uses a radioactive substance to detect the level of dopamine transporters (DaT) in the brain: these transporters pump the important neurotransmitter dopamine out of the synapse and into the cell liquid, and their excess can lead to a depletion of dopamine. As the examining neurologist explained, in cases of loss of 70 per cent of dopaminergic neurons, new synapses connect striatal neurons and more dopamine receptors compensate for the loss. Clinical symptoms of Parkinson's usually appear beyond an 80 per cent loss, but a DaTscan detects it even at 30 to 40 per cent.
45. This form of listening was a kind of 'ethnopsychiatry'. The term was coined by a Haitian psychologist named Louis Mars, and taken up in 1954 by Georges Devereux, a French anthropologist who became a psychoanalyst and combined both practices in his exploration of how healing takes place within a culturally embedded, socially specific practice, rather than on the basis of a theory. See Georges Bloch, *Les Origines culturelles de Georges Devereux et la naissance de l'ethnopsychiatrie*, http://www.ethnopsychiatrie.net/actu/GBGD.htm
46. See my *Passions and Tempers*: pp. 16–17 on Asclepios, and pp. 73–80 on medicine and faith in the early Middle Ages.

47. Sigmund Freud, tr. James Strachey, *The Interpretation of Dreams*, vol. 4 of *The Standard Edition of the Complete Psychological Works of Sigmund Freud* (1958) (London: Penguin, 1976), pp. 164–5.

48. Abd Ar Rahman bin Muhammed ibn Khaldun, *Muqaddimah*, tr. Franz Rosenthal, 'Sixth Prefatory Discussion: The various types of human beings who have supernatural perception either through natural disposition or through exercise, preceded by a discussion of inspiration and dream visions'.

49. See Tanya Marie Luhrmann et al., 'Culture and Hallucinations: Overview and Future Directions', *Schizophrenia Bulletin*, 40, 2014, supp. 4, pp. S213–20: 'An ethnographic approach to hallucinations therefore becomes essential in understanding how members of particular societies identify and understand sensory events that would be recognized by secular observers as hallucinations and how they distinguish between unusual sensory events they regard as appropriate and those they identify as signs of illness' (p. S213). And: 'the evidence suggests that the voice-hearing experience is deeply shaped by local patterns of understanding the self, the mind, and the fundamental nature of reality' (p. S217).

50. See Ariel Levy, 'The Drug of Choice for the Age of Kale', *New Yorker*, 5 September 2016. The potentially therapeutic effects of psychotropic substances are now being seriously investigated. See the noted volume by Michael Pollan, *How to Change Your Mind: What the New Science of Psychedelics Teaches Us About Consciousness, Dying, Addiction, Depression, and Transcendence* (New York, NY: Penguin, 2018).

51. British psychotherapist and theorist Donald W. Winnicott writes in 'The Concept of a Healthy Individual', a lecture he gave in 1967, reprinted in the collection *Home is Where We Start From* (London and New York, NY: Penguin, 1986), : 'I have tried to work out where cultural experience is located, and I have tentatively made this formulation: that it starts *in the potential space between the child and the mother when experience has produced in the child a high degree of confidence in*

the mother, that she will not fail to be there if suddenly needed', p. 36. That same year, he pursued the topic in his essay entitled 'The Location of Cultural Experience', reprinted in *Playing and Reality* (1971) (London and New York, NY: Routledge, 2005), where he offers this: 'The place where cultural experience is located is in the *potential space* between the individual and the environment (originally the object). The same can be said of playing. Cultural experience begins with creative living first manifested in play' (p. 135).

Chapter 5: Appearances

1. The research on this is plentiful. See for instance Davangere P. Davanand, 'Olfactory Identification Deficits, Cognitive Decline, and Dementia in Older Adults', *American Journal of Geriatric Psychiatry*, 24: 12, December 2016, pp. 1,151–7.
2. The syndrome was thus baptized by Franco-Swiss neurologist Georges de Morsier, in 1967. See Tiffany Jan and Jorge del Castillo, 'Visual Hallucinations: Charles Bonnet Syndrome', *Western Journal of Emergency Medicine*, 13: 6, December 2012.
3. Bonnet remains known for his work on the parthenogenesis of aphids, which breed very fast, and in part asexually, females giving birth to female nymphs.
4. John Locke, *An Essay Concerning Human Understanding* (1700) (Oxford, Clarendon Press, 1975), Book 2, chs 1–3, pp. 104–22.
5. Charles Bonnet, *Essai analytique sur les facultés de l'âme* (Copenhagen: Frères Philibert, 1760).
6. Sacks, *Hallucinations*, pp. 5–8.
7. See an essay on the history of the condition by neurologist Frederick E. Lepore, 'When Seeing Is Not Believing', Dana Foundation, *Cerebrum*, 1 April 2002, https://dana.org/article/when-seeing-is-not-believing/
8. See D. H. ffytche et al., 'The Anatomy of Conscious Vision: An fMRI Study of Visual Hallucinations', *Nature Neuroscience*, 1: 8, December 1998, pp. 738–42. Oliver Sacks refers to this

study in his pages on Charles Bonnet Syndrome in *Hallucinations*, pp. 23–4: 'When there were colored hallucinations, there was activation of areas in the visual cortex associated with color construction; when there were facial hallucinations of a sketchlike or cartoonlike character, there was activation in the fusiform gyrus' (p. 23). Sacks writes in *Hallucinations* that ffytche et al., 'observed, moreover, a clear distinction between normal visual imagination and actual hallucination – thus, imagining a colored object, for example, did not activate the V4 area, while a colored hallucination did. Such findings confirm that, not only subjectively but physiologically, hallucinations are unlike imagination and much more like perceptions. Writing of hallucinations in 1760, Bonnet said, "The mind would not be able to tell apart vision from reality." The work of ffytche and his colleagues shows that the brain does not distinguish them, either.'

9. Miriam Rothschild (1908–2005) was known in Britain for her work on flea locomotion and reproduction; she also did much research on the relationship of parasites with their hosts, of plants with insects and butterflies, and so on.

10. See David P. Reichert et al., 'Charles Bonnet Syndrome: Evidence for a Generative Model in the Cortex?', *PLoS Computational Biology*, 18 July 2013, 9: 7, and Philip Corlett et al., 'Hallucinations and Strong Priors', *Trends in Cognitive Sciences*, February 2019, vol. 23, no. 2, pp. 114–27: 'in response to low-level impairments, homeostatic mechanisms stabilize network activity levels such that hallucinations arise when input is lacking, consistent with the observation that de-afferented cortex becomes hyper-excitable; we argue this reflects the imposition of explanatory priors on noisy inputs' (p. 122), and: 'Indeed, visual processing, while integrated, possesses dissociable streams for inferences about exteroceptive, interoceptive, and proprioceptive states (i.e., actions)' (p. 119).

11. See Olaf Blanke et al., 'Audio-Visual Sensory Deprivation Degrades Visuo-Tactile Peripersonal Space', *Consciousness and Cognition*, 61, May 2018, pp. 61–75.

12. Dysexecutive syndrome might be a simplifying and even falsifying misnomer. In 1995, Donald T. Stuss et al., in 'A Multidisciplinary Approach to Anterior Attentional Functions', *Annals of the New York Academy of Sciences*, 15 December 1995, 769, pp. 191–211, had proposed that there was no such thing as a dysexecutive syndrome because there was no central executive in the first place: 'If we are correct that there is no central executive, neither can there be a dysexecutive syndrome. The frontal lobes (in anatomical terms) or the supervisory system (in cognitive terms) do not function (in physiological terms) as a simple (inexplicable) homunculus. Monitoring, energizing, inhibition, etc. – these are processes that exist at many levels of the brain, including those more posterior 'automatic' processes. Owing to their extensive reciprocal connections with virtually all other brain regions, the frontal lobes may be unique in the quality of the processes that have evolved, and perhaps in the level of processing which might be labelled "executive"' or "supervisory"' (p. 206). With Michael P. Alexander, Stuss refers to this paragraph in 'Is There a Dysexecutive Syndrome?', *Philosophical Transactions of the Royal Society B*, 2007, 362, pp. 901–15. They conclude: 'The functioning of what has been called the central executive or supervisory system can be explained by the flexible assembly of these processes in response to context, complexity and intention over real time into different networks within the frontal regions, and between frontal and posterior regions. There is no overarching supervisory system – no "ghost in the machine" – that is higher in the hierarchy' (p. 911).

13. See Hugo D. Critchley, 'The Human Cortex Responds to an Interoceptive Challenge', *Proceedings of the National Academy of Sciences*, 27 April 2004, 101: 17, pp. 6,333–4. See Damasio, *Descartes's Error*, ch. 4, 'In Colder Blood', pp. 52–79: p. 70; idem., *The Feeling of What Happens*, pp. 41, 267–74; idem, *Self Comes to Mind*, pp. 103, 283–4, 310.

14. Fritz Heinrich Lewy (1885–1950), a German-American neurologist, had discovered in 1912 clumps of proteins in the

brains of patients with behavioural and cognitive impediments. These clusters of proteins were named 'Lewy bodies' by the Russian neurologist Konstantin Tretiakoff, just a few years after Lewy had first found them in patients with Parkinson's Disease, in the substantia nigra area of the brain. One of the proteins that composes Lewy Bodies was later identified as α-synuclein. The protein is essential to synaptic communication between neurons, and the effect of these clumps was to disable the communication of neurons and disrupt neurotransmitters. This is what occurs in Parkinson's Disease – itself named by Charcot after James Parkinson, who had described what he called 'the shaking palsy'. See Kelly Del Tredici et al., '100 years of Lewy Pathology', *Nature Reviews Neurology*, 9 January 2013, pp. 13–24. On hallucinations in LBD, see Stefania Pezzoli et al., 'Structural and Functional Neuroimaging of Visual Hallucinations in Lewy Body Disease: A Systematic Literature Review', *Brain Science*, 7: 84, 2017.

15. The main proteins to play a role in AD are tau and β-amyloid.
16. For information about DaTscans, see above, n. 44 to ch. 4.
17. See Annachiara Cagnin et al., 'Sleep-wake Profile in Dementia with Lewy Bodies, Alzheimer's Disease, and Normal Aging', *Journal of Alzheimer's Disease*, 55: 4, 2017, pp. 1,529–36.
18. See Daniel C. Mograbi and Robin G. Morris, 'On the Relation among Mood, Apathy, and Anosognosia in Alzheimer's Disease', *Journal of the International Neuropsychological Society*, 20: 1, January 2014, pp. 2–7. They report here that 'Depressed mood is found to be associated with less anosognosia, while greater apathy is associated with more anosognosia' (abstract).
19. Cagnin et al., Sleep-wake Profile in Dementia' (2017). For a review of studies of circadian clock disturbances in AD, see Johannes Thome et al., 'The Circadian System in Alzheimer's Disease: Disturbances, Mechanisms, and Opportunities', *Biological Psychiatry*, 74: 5, 2013, pp. 333–9: 'There is considerable evidence that disturbances of sleep–wake cycles

are related to alterations in the suprachiasmatic nucleus (SCN), the master circadian pacemaker.'

20. For analyses of how the perception of time is a function of interoception, see Marc Wittmann, 'Embodied Time: The Experience of Time, the Body, and the Self', in Valtteri Arstila and Dan Lloyd, eds, *Subjective Time* (Cambridge, MA and London: MIT Press, 2014); Marc Wittmann and Karin Meissner, 'The Embodiment of Time: How Interoception Shapes the Perception of Time', in Tsakiris and de Preester, eds, *The Interoceptive Mind*, pp. 63–79; Giuseppe Riva et al., 'Feel the Time. Time Perception as a Function of Interoceptive Processing', *Frontiers in Human Neuroscience*, 12: 74, March 2018.

21. According to the World Health Organization, about 50 million people worldwide live with dementia, and the number rises constantly (see https://www.who.int/news-room/fact-sheets/detail/dementia). But if age is a major risk factor for the development of neurodegenerative disease, it is not identical with it. There are dementias that can begin when one is relatively young. And the term itself has a historically ambivalent status: in the eighteenth century, 'dementia' denoted any intellectual deficit, regardless of age – eventually covering also what we today name schizophrenia (see below, n. 9 to ch. 6). See also Frédéric Assal, 'History of Dementia', in Julien Bogousslavsky et al., eds, *A History of Neuropsychology* (Basel: Karger, 2019), Frontiers of Neurology and Neuroscience, 44, pp. 118–26.

22. Shakespeare, *The Winter's Tale*, Act 4, Scene 4, ll. 398–404.

23. Assal, 'History of Dementia', in Bogousslavsky et al., eds, *A History of Neuropsychology*. See also Stavros J. Baloyannis, 'Galen as Neuroscientist and Neurophilosopher', *Encephalos*, 53, 2016, pp. 1–10: p. 7.

24. See my *Passions and Tempers*.

25. The actual pathologization of mental decline, and the identification of processes involved in it, started only with the advent of modern neuroscience in the late nineteenth century, with figures such as Aloïs Alzheimer or Emil Redlich, who

started to identify the biology of dementias, including the protein tangles in the disease to which Alzheimer gave his name. See Aloïs Alzheimer, 'Über eine eigenartige Erkrankung der Hirnrinde', *Allgemeine Zeitschrift für Psychiatrie und psychisch-gerichtliche Medizin*, 64, 1907, pp. 146–8. See also Michel Goedert, 'Oskar Fischer and the Study of Dementia', *Brain*, 132: 4, April 2009, pp. 1,102–11. And see Finger, *Origins of Neuroscience*, pp. 351–5.

26. See my 'Thoughts Made Visible', *Lapham's Quarterly*, 9: 1, Winter 2018, *States of Mind*, pp. 191–8, https://www.laphamsquarterly.org/states-mind/thoughts-made-visible: 'But it is functional imaging that has transformed neuroscientific and neuropsychological research. It registers minute metabolic changes, enabling researchers to pinpoint which parts of the brain are most saliently at work on specific tasks compared to other parts, giving a real-time picture of cerebral activity. In fact, by 1890, a number of researchers, including William James, had already correctly reported that variations in blood flow in the brain correspond to neuronal activity – a phenomenon called neurovascular coupling – and this is what functional scans make use of. PET scans – positron-emission tomography – work by tracing injected radioactive substances to see how they bind to brain receptors. So do SPECT scans, single-photon emission computed tomography. Then in 1990 the fMRI – the functional version of MRI – was introduced. It is much less invasive than PET and often more precise in terms of spatial resolution, with the caveat that temporal resolution remains a problem, since cerebral activity is far faster than the machine' (p. 196).

27. See Morris and Mograbi, 'Anosognosia, Autobiographical Memory and Self-knowledge in Alzheimer's Disease' (2013), and, above, n. 4 to ch. 3.

28. Damasio, *Self Comes to Mind*, pp. 230–1, and pp. 229–33 on AD specifically; on the 'three stages of self – protoself, core self, autobiographical self', pp. 181 ff. On the core self, see above, n. 17 to ch. 3.

Chapter 6: Guilty as Charged

1. See Yaakov Stern, 'Cognitive Reserve in Ageing and Alzheimer's Disease', *Lancet Neurology*, 11: 11, November 2012, pp. 1,006–12.

2. See for instance Alfredo Berardelli et al., 'Pathophysiology of Bradykinesia in Parkinson's Disease', *Brain*, 124: 11, November 2001, pp. 2,131–46. Bradykinesia is a so-called extrapyramidal symptom – involuntary movements that include all manner of tremor – and can be iatrogenic, that is, caused by medication. They are a well-known side-effect of the anti-psychotic treatments such as the neuroleptics Eric was taking, but, in his case, they could have been caused by the neurodegenerative disease itself.

3. The pioneers of L-Dopa treatment for Parkinson's are Arvid Carlsson, Oleh Hornykiewicz, George Cotzias, and Melvin Yahr. See Andrew J. Lees, Eduardo Tolosa, and C. Warren Olanow, 'Four Pioneers of L-dopa Treatment: Arvid Carlsson, Oleh Hornykiewicz, George Cotzias, and Melvin Yahr', *Movement Disorders*, 30: 1, January 2015. See also Alison Abbott, 'Levodopa: The Story So Far', *Nature*, 466, 25 August 2010, pp. S6–7.

4. Oliver Sacks, *Awakenings* (1973) (New York: HarperCollins, 1990/London: Picador, 1991). L-Dopa is a precursor of dopamine that can traverse the brain–blood barrier, and so is prescribed to augment the circulation of dopamine, whose deficiency accompanies a large number of neurological troubles, including Parkinson's and LBD. In some of its symptoms – notably sleep disturbance and dysexecutive syndrome – LBD can indeed resemble the late stages of Parkinson's Disease, insofar as both affect the dopaminergic system. See for instance Juebin Huang, 'Dementia with Lewy Bodies and Parkinson Disease Dementia', *Merck Manual* (Professional version), December 2019, https://www.merckmanuals.com/professional/neurologic-disorders/delirium-and-dementia/dementia-with-lewy-bodies-and-parkinson-disease-dementia

5. See Dolores Malaspina et al., 'Schizoaffective Disorder in the DSM-5', *Schizophrenia Research*, 150: 1, October 2013, pp. 21–5.

6. See Berrios and Porter, eds, *A History of Clinical Psychiatry*: 'It is an ironic unintended consequence of modern medicine's efficacy that the pharmaceuticals employed may ocasionally serve to blunt the distinction between disease and medicine – or in other words, "iatrogenesis" has become an intrinsic feature of contemporary medicine' (p. 117). See also for instance Chiara Rafanelli and Giovanni Fava, 'Iatrogenic Factors in Psychopathology', *Psychotherapy and Psychosomatics*, 88: 1, 2019, pp. 129–40.

7. See Vasilios C. Constantinides et al., 'Corticobasal Degeneration and Corticobasal Syndrome: A Review', *Clinical Parkinsonism & Related Disorders*, 1, 2019, pp. 66–71.

8. See Charles Raymond Lake, 'Hypothesis: Grandiosity and Guilt Cause Paranoia; Paranoid Schizophrenia is a Psychotic Mood Disorder; A Review', *Schizophrenia Bulletin*, 34: 6, November 2008, pp. 1,151–62.

9. *DSM 5: Diagnostic and Statistic Manual of Mental Disorders* (American Psychiatric Association, 2013), https://dsm. psychiatryonline.org/doi/full/10.1176/appi. books.9780890425596.dsm02, under 'Schizophrenia Spectrum and Other Psychotic Disorders'.

10. Sigmund Freud, trans. James Strachey, *Introductory Lectures on Psychoanalysis* (1917) (London: Pelican, 1973), Lecture 16, 'Psychoanalysis and Psychiatry': 'You will grant that there is nothing in the nature of psychiatric work which could be opposed to psychanalytic work. What is opposed to psychoanalysis is not psychiatry but psychiatrists. Psychoanalysis is related to psychiatry approximately as histology is to anatomy: the one studies the external forms of the organs, the other studies their construction out of tissues and cells' (p. 294). See also Yohan Trichet, 'The Freudian Clinic of the Onset of Psychosis', *Recherches en psychanalyse* 2011/2, pp. 197–205.

11. On Emil Kraepelin, see above, n. 19 to ch. 2. See also Appignanesi, *Mad, Bad and Sad*, pp. 203–4.

12. Eugen Bleuler (1857–1939) 'applied to psychosis the mechanisms that Freud had recognized in the field of neurosis', as notes Thomas G. Dalzell, 'Eugen Bleuler 150: Bleuler's Reception of Freud', *History of Psychiatry*, 18: 4, pp. 471–82: p. 472. See 'Eugen Bleuler's Dementia Praecox or the Group of Schizophrenias (1911): A Centenary Appreciation and Reconsideration', *Schizophrenia Bulletin*, 37: 3, May 2011, pp. 471–9. See also Makari, *Revolution in Mind*, p. 183.

13. Initially, schizophrenia had referred to 'hebephrenia', yet another term used by an earlier psychiatrist, Ewald Hecker, to name a rapidly degenerative condition that afflicted adolescents. French psychiatrist Augustin Morel used 'dementia praecox' before Kraepelin adopted it. See Emil Kraepelin, *Lectures on Clinical Psychiatry* (3rd English edition of the translation from the German: 1913). And see Appignanesi, *Mad, Bad and Sad*.

14. See Lena Palaniyappan and Peter F Liddle, 'Does the Salience Network Play a Cardinal Role in Psychosis? An Emerging Hypothesis of Insular Dysfunction', *Journal of Psychiatry and Neuroscience*, 37: 1, January 2012, pp. 17–27.

15. See in this regard the incisive work of philosopher Robert C. Solomon, in particular his *True to Our Feelings: What Our Emotions Are Really Telling Us* (Oxford and New York, NY: Oxford University Press, 2007).

16. See Darian Leader, *What is Madness?* (London: Hamish Hamilton, 2011), pp. 137–40.

17. The school of neuropsychoanalysis founded in the 1990s by neuropsychologist and psychoanalyst Mark Solms is one important exception to this, albeit within the realm of theoretical research. A notable, concerted and systematic *clinical* effort to apply psychotherapeutic techniques specifically to the treatment of psychoses, and to understand psychopathology in its 'existential' dimension, was that of the US-based Italians Silvano Arieti (1914–81), a specialist of

schizophrenia and Gaetano Benedetti (1920–2013), originally a neurologist, and the Swiss psychiatrist Christian Müller. Benedetti was convinced one could 'only understand psychopathology with a psychotherapeutic gaze': see Martin Reca, 'Présentation de l'approche psychothérapique pour les patients schizophrènes de Gaetano Benedetti: à propos de la réédition en France de son œuvre principale, *La Psychothérapie de la schizophrénie. Existence et transfert* (Érès, 2010)', *L'Information psychiatrique*, 1: 87, 2011, pp. 31–6, https://www. cairn.info/revue-l-information-psychiatrique-2011-1-page-31. htm. Together the three men founded the still extant ISPS, or International Society for Psychological and Social Approaches to Psychosis (formerly, International Society for the Psychological Treatments of the Schizophrenias and Other Psychoses). As noted by Brian Koehler in 'Interview with Gaetano Benedetti, M.D.', *Journal of the American Academy of Psychoanalysis and Dynamic Psychiatry*, 31, 2003: 'The Schizophrenic Person and the Benefits of the Psychotherapies – Seeking a PORT in the Storm', Benedetti 'and his younger colleague in the field of schizophrenia, Dr Maurizio Peciccia, understand the illness to be the result of an interaction between possible neurobiological vulnerabilities, overwhelming affects, and a self lacking cohesion and integration. Specifically, they characterize the core psychological deficit in schizophrenia to be a deintegration of the separate and symbiotic selves of the patient, resulting in the oscillation between pathological symbiosis with the world and a defensive autistic-like retreat from object relations' (pp. 75–87). For a similar effort at bridging biology and psychology, see Filipe Arantes-Gonçalves, João Gama Marques, and Diogo Telles-Correia, 'Bleuler's Psychopathological Perspective on Schizophrenia Delusions: Towards New Tools in Psychotherapy Treatment', *Frontiers in Psychiatry*, 17 July 2018.

18. See Philippe Rochat, 'The Ontogeny of Human Self-Consciousness', *Current Directions in Psychological Science*, 2016, pp 1–6. Children typically acquire a social self-consciousness

by the age of two, as Darwin had observed – the very age at which they pass the so-called mirror test: see above, n.1 to ch. 1. Rochat writes: 'Unlike other animals, human infants who pass the mirror mark test show social emotions such as embarrassment, marked inhibition, pride, or acting out . . . What they recognize in the mirror is not only their embodied self but also their public self, that is, how others might see them. From this point on, social referencing is not only outward, but also inward' (p. 3).

19. See in particular Bernard Williams, *Shame and Necessity* (Berkeley, Los Angeles, London: University of California Press, 1993), pp. 88–102. There is much research on the operations and functions of guilt within social psychology, in relation to developmental psychology. See for instance Amrisha Vaish, 'The Prosocial Functions of Early Social Emotions: The Case of Guilt', *Current Opinion in Psychology*, 20, April 2018, pp. 25–9; Amrisha Vaish, Malinda Carpenter, and Michael Tomasello, 'Young Children's Responses to Guilt Displays', *Developmental Psychology*, 47: 5, September 2011, pp. 1,248–62.

20. Freud, trans. Strachey, *Introductory Lectures on Psychoanalysis* (1917), Lecture 21, 'The Development of the Libido and the Sexual Organizations', p. 375.

21. See Melanie Klein, *Love, Guilt, and Reparation, and Other Works, 1921–1945* (New York, NY: The Free Press, 1975); Michael Lewis, 'The Development of Guilt as Repair in Childhood', https://emotionresearcher.com/the-development-of-guilt-as-repair-in-childhood/ Klein dated the onset of an emotion of guilt to early infancy, a notion that is not borne out by infant research such as that conducted by Philippe Rochat (see above, n. 16, and n. 1 to ch. 1).

22. See Paul C. Fletcher and Chris D Frith, 'Perceiving Is Believing: A Bayesian Approach to Explaining the Positive Symptoms of Schizophrenia', *Nature Reviews Neuroscience*, 10: 1, January 2009, pp. 48–58, where they argue that 'a common mechanism, involving minimization of prediction error, may

underlie perception and inference, and that a disruption in this mechanism may cause both abnormal perceptions (hallucinations) and abnormal beliefs (delusions)' (p. 48).

23. Dimitris Bolis and Leonhard Schilbach, '"Through Others We Become Ourselves": The Dialectics of Predictive Coding and Active Inference', *Behavioral and Brain Sciences*, 43, 2020, e93.

24. Freud, *Neurosis and Psychosis*, in *Complete Works*: 2 (1924), pp. 250–4, Freud also sees an affinity between dreaming and psychosis.

25. Donald Winnicott, *Playing and Reality* (1971) (London: Routledge, 1991), passim: pp. 13–19. See James Barnes, 'For Donald Winnicott, the Psyche is not Inside Us but Between Us', *Psyche*, May 2020, https://psyche.co/ideas/for-donald-winnicott-the-psyche-is-not-inside-us-but-between-us. Barnes believes that Freud's view of a dichotomy between the self as subject independent from, and even in opposition to an 'objective' world has been as misguided as Cartesian dualism. By contrast, he writes, Winnicott gave us a more sensible view: 'Experience of the world and others is the primary given, and minds – rather than traversing an existing separation – are in a certain sense responsible for creating it. Effectively, this is an inversion of Freud's dualistic model.' Freud was not as dualistic as Barnes asserts, but the emphasis Winnicott puts on the 'parent-child dyad' is indeed a major shift.

26. See Vittorio Gallese, 'A New Take on Intersubjectivity', in Massimo Ammaniti and Vittorio Gallese, eds, *The Birth of Intersubjectivity: Psychodynamics, Neurobiology, and the Self* (New York, NY and London: W. W. Norton, 2014), pp. 1–25. See Bolis and Schilbach, '"I Interact Therefore I Am"'.

27. See primarily Fotopoulou and Tsakiris, 'Mentalizing Homeostasis' (2017), where the authors argue that 'even some of the most minimal aspects of selfhood, namely the feeling qualities associated with being an embodied subject, are fundamentally shaped by embodied interactions with other people in early infancy and beyond' (abstract). (See also n. 19

to ch. 1, above.) As I wrote regarding their argument in 'The Interoceptive Turn' (2019): 'Our capacity to modulate affect begins with the carer attending to the infant's embodied needs. Out of the processing of sensorimotor signals initially integrated into a basic, minimal or core self arise what they call "embodied mentalisations" that progressively lead to our ability to form a boundary between self and other – a process that cannot happen in isolation. It is necessarily in relation to others that we acquire a sense of self, which develops in this embodied interoceptive way from infancy on. We sustain a constant sense of selfhood in dynamic relation to and distinction from others, and, in turn, our ability to form a boundary between self and other is a function of our ability to feel our embodied selves from within – this is the important novelty of their claim. An unformed or badly formed boundary can translate into psychiatric pathologies.' See also: Anna Ciaunica, 'Introduction: The Relational Self: Basic Forms of Self-Awareness', *Topoi*, 39, 20 January 2020, pp. 501–7; Manos Tsakiris, 'The Multisensory Basis of the self: From Body to Identity to Others', *Quarterly Journal of Experimental Biology*, 70: 4, 2017, pp. 597–609; Andrea Serino et al., 'Bodily Ownership and Self-location: Components of Bodily Self-consciousness', *Consciousness and Cognition*, 22, 2013, pp. 1,239–52; Vivien Ainley, Matthew Apps, Aikaterini Fotopoulou, Manos Tsakiris, '"Bodily Precision": A Predictive Coding Account of Individual Differences in Interoceptive Accuracy', *Philosophical Transactions of the Royal Society B*, 371, 2016. 0003, 2016; Seth and Friston, 'Active Interoceptive Inference' (2016); Lisa Feldman Barrett, Karen S. Quigley, and Paul Hamilton, 'An Active Inference Theory of Allostasis and Interoception in Depression', *Philosophical Transactions of the Royal Society B*, 371, 2016. 0011, 2016: 'we hypothesize that interoceptive predictions are part of every concept that is learned and constructed, and categorization via concepts is the prime computation by which the emotion regulation process, cognitive reappraisal, takes place' (p. 8).

28. Damasio, *Self Comes to Mind*, and see above, n. 27 to ch. 6. See also Vittorio Gallese and Corrado Sinigaglia, 'The Bodily Self as Power for Action', *Neuropsychologia*, 48: 3, February 2010, pp. 746–55. For the notion of a 'minimal self', see especially the work of Dan Zahavi, and, above, n. 1 to ch. 3. And see Anna Ciaunica and Laura Crucianelli, 'Minimal Self-Awareness: From Within a Developmental Perspective', *Journal of Consciousness Studies* 26: 3–4, 2019, pp. 207–26.

29. See Aikaterini Fotopoulou and Anna Ciaunica, 'The Touched Self: Psychological and Philosophical Perspectives on Proximal Intersubjectivity and the Self', in Christoph Durt, Thomas Fuchs, and Christian Tewes, *Embodiment, Enaction, and Culture: Investigating the Constitution of the Shared World* (Cambridge, MA and London: MIT Press, 2017).

30. See Damasio's accounts of this: above, n. 19 to ch. 1. And see Jaak Panksepp, *Affective Neuroscience: The Foundations of Human and Animal Emotions* (Oxford and New York, NY: Oxford University Press, 1998), the first chapter of which opens with: 'Our emotional feelings reflect our ability to subjectively experience certain states of the nervous system' (p. 9).

31. See Maurizio Peciccia et al., 'Constructing the Sense of Self in Psychosis Using the Amniotic Therapy: A Single Case Study', *Psychosis: Psychological, Social and Integrative Approaches*, June 2019: 'Psychosis has been conceptualized from the psychoanalytical perspective as a disturbance in the embodied self and its boundaries, namely a disruption of the preverbal sense of oneself as a cohesive, volitional, bounded entity' (p. 1).

32. See Seth, Suzuki, and Critchley, 'An Interoceptive Predictive Coding Model of Conscious Presence', (2012).

33. See Olga Pollatos et al., 'Reduced Perception of Bodily Signals in Anorexia Nervosa', *Eating Behaviors*, 9: 4, December 2008, pp. 381-8; Beate Herbert et al., 'Interoception across Modalities: On the Relationship between Cardiac Awareness and the Sensitivity for Gastric Functions', *PLoS One*, 7: 5, May 2012; Kate Tchanturia, Catherine Stewart, and Emma Kinnaird, 'Interoception in Anorexia Nervosa: Exploring

Associations With Alexithymia and Autistic Traits', *Frontiers of Psychiatry*, 21 February 2020.

34. See Martina Ardizzi et al., 'Interoception and Positive Symptoms in Schizophrenia', *Frontiers in Human Neuroscience*, 10: 379, 27 July 2016: 'the attribution of feelings and sensations to one's own body presupposes an intact basic sense of self' (p. 2), precisely what is amiss in psychotic patients. 'Overall, it seems that high self-opinion or focused attention on explicit aspects of these are associated to increased sensitivity to the internal signals of the body. Drawing from this evidence, we speculated that while interoception might contribute to boost the explicit self-representation in healthy controls, it might contribute to a pathologically hyperbolic explicit self representation in schizophrenia patients, characterized by a distorted sense of self. Grandiosity and grandiose delusions among schizophrenia patients, as well as narcissism traits in healthy participants, are indeed frequently described as defensive compensations against failures, dissatisfactions with life and traumatic events . . . From this point of view, grandiosity and grandiose delusions might be protective also against the altered basic sense of self characterizing schizophrenia patients with higher sensibility to inner bodily sensations. The loss of *"the circumference centre"* might find its compensation by artificially building an explicit over-extended self, particularly among patients who are more in tune with their own internal bodily signals' (p. 7).

35. See above, n. 17.

36. See for instance Elena A. Bondarenko et al., 'Genetic Factors in Major Depression Disease', *Frontiers of Psychiatry*, 9: 334, 2018; Alex S. F. Kwong et al., 'Genetic and Environmental Risk Factors Associated with Trajectories of Depression Symptoms From Adolescence to Young Adulthood', *Jama Network Open*, 2: 6, July 2019.

37. See Laura Marsh, 'Depression and Parkinson's Disease: Current Knowledge', *Current Neurology and Neuroscience Reports*, 13: 12, December 2013: 'It is generally accepted that clinically

significant depressive disturbances occur in 40–50 % of patients with PD. As such, depression is one of the most frequently reported neuropsychiatric disturbances in PD' (p. 409).

38. William Styron, *Darkness Visible* (New York, NY: Random House, 1990). Memoirs about depression have multiplied since, with such works as Elizabeth Wurtzel, *Prozac Nation: Young and Depressed in America* (New York, NY: Riverhead, 1995); Kay Redfield Jamison, *An Unquiet Mind: A Memoir of Moods and Madness* (New York, NY: Vintage, 1996); Andrew Solomon, *The Noonday Demon: An Atlas of Depression* (New York, NY: Simon & Schuster, 2001); Céline Curiol, *Un Quinze Août à Paris: histoire d'une dépression* (Arles: Actes Sud, 2016); Daphne Merkin, *This Close to Happy: A Reckoning with Depression* (New York, NY: Farrar, Straus & Giroux, 2017), and many more.

39. See my *Passions and Tempers*, pp. 155–70.

40. Kraepelin's section on 'maniac-depressive insanity' is section 2 of vol. 3 of his 1913 *Psychiatrie*. A French translation appeared the same year in *Revue des Sciences Psychologiques*, re-issued as a book on its centennial as *La Folie maniaque-dépressive* (Paris: Jérôme Millon, 2013) And see Porter, *Madness*, pp. 183–7.

41. Editorial, 'Bipolar Disorder: At the Extremes', *The Lancet*, 381: 9878, 11 May 2013, p. 1,597.

42. For a rich history of this symptomatology, and of the wide nosological and semantic range it gave rise to, see Berrios and Porter, eds, *A History of Clinical Psychiatry*, ch. 15, 'Mood Disorders', pp. 384–420.

43. See my 'As a Lute Out of Tune' (2013) and, above, n. 11 to ch. 2. There is a vast literature on melancholy, and on its history.

44. See Lionel Laborie, *Enlightening Enthusiasm: Prophecy and Religious Experience in Early Eighteenth-Century England* (Manchester: Manchester University Press, 2015).

45. See David S. Lovejoy, *Religious Enthusiasm in the New World* (Cambridge, MA and London: Harvard University Press, 2014).

46. John Moore, *Of Religious Melancholy: A Sermon Preach'd Before the Queen at White-Hall, March the 6th, 1691/2*. By the Right Reverend Father in God, John, Lord Bishop of Norwich. Published by Her Majesty's Special Command. See also Julius H. Rubin, *Religious Melancholy and Protestant Experience in America* (Oxford and New York, NY: Oxford University Press, 1994), p. 88.

47. Richard Blackmore, *A Treatise of the Spleen and Vapours, Or, Hypocondriacal and Hysterical Affections, With Three Discourses on the Nature and Cure of the Cholick, Melancholy, and Palsies* (London: J. Pemberton, 1725), Preface, p. vii. Blackmore was also a mediocre poet and writer of politically oriented epics, mocked for his leaden style by his contemporaries, most famously – and bitingly – by Jonathan Swift in his *On Poetry* (1733), and in *Verses on Sir Richard Blackmore*.

48. Soeur Jeanne des Anges, *Autobiographie d'une hystérique possédée, d'après le manuscrit inédit de la bibliothèque de Tours, annoté et publié par les Drs Gabriel Legué et Gilles de La Tourette. Préface de M. le professeur Charcot . . .*' (Paris: Progrès médical, 1886), catalogue.bnf.fr/ark:/12148/cb30650688b

49. See Ephraim Radner, 'Early Modern Jansenism', in Ulrich L. Lehner, Richard Alfred Muller, and A. G. Roeber, eds, *The Oxford Handbook of Early Modern Theology, 1600–1800* (Oxford and New York, NY: Oxford University Press, 2016), pp. 436–50.

50. See Adrien Borel, 'Les Convulsionnaires et le diacre Pâris', *L'Evolution psychiatrique*, 4, 1935, pp. 3–24, http://www.histoiredelafolie.fr/psychiatrie-neurologie/les-convulsionnaires-du-cimetiere-de-la-saint-medard-et-le-diacre-paris-par-adrien-borel-1935. See also Nicolas Lyon-Caen, 'Un "Saint de nouvelle fabrique": le diacre Paris (1690–1727), le jansénisme et la bonneterie parisienne', *Annales: Histoire, Sciences Sociales*, 2010: 3, pp. 613–42.

51. These *Pensées* were published posthumously, as *Pensées de M. Pascal sur la religion et sur quelques autres sujets, qui ont été trouvées après sa mort parmi ses papiers* (Paris, 1669).

52. Pascal, *Pensées*, p. 434. Here in the English translation by W. F. Trotter (New York, NY: E. P. Dutton, 1958).

53. For an analysis of Pascal's complex relation to Jansenism, see Albert R. Jonsen and Stephen Toulmin, *The Abuse of Casuistry: A History of Moral Reasoning* (Berkeley and Los Angeles, CA, London: University of California Press, 1988), ch. 12, 'Casuistry Confounded: Pascal's Critique', pp. 231–49.

Chapter 7: Hold My Hand

1. See for instance E. Kocagoncu et al., 'Evidence and Implications of Abnormal Predictive Coding in Dementia', arXiv preprint, https://arxiv.org/ftp/arxiv/papers/2006/2006.06311.pdf

2. See Camilla N. Clark and Jason D. Warren, 'Music, Memory and Mechanisms in Alzheimer's Disease', and Jörn-Henrik Jacobsen et al., 'Why Musical Memory can be Preserved in Advanced Alzheimer's Disease', both in *Brain*, 138: 8, August 2015, respectively pp. 2,122–5 and pp. 2,438–50. Oliver Sacks devoted the last chapter of his *Musicophilia: Tales of Music and the Brain* (New York, NY and Toronto: Knopf, 2007), pp. 335–47, to the preservation in dementia of the musical sense in connection to that of affect, and to the various musical therapies that can be used to help patients.

3. See Elisabeth M. J. Foncke and Marina A. J. de Koning-Tijssen, 'Myoclonus-Dystonia/Essential Myoclonus', *Encyclopedia of Movement Disorders* (Elsevier, 2010), pp. 248–51.

4. The extrapyramidal, as opposed to the pyramidal system – both a part of the motor system, along with the cerebellar system – is thus called because its tracts don't traverse the 'pyramids' of the medulla, that vital part of the brainstem which regulates heartbeat, breathing, blood pressure, and more. The extrapyramidal system is evolutionarily very ancient – we share it with the first creatures endowed with motion – and it modulates reflex responses, directed movement, posture, and so on.

5. Damasio, *The Strange Order of Things*, pp. 82–116.
6. *DSM 5*, see online https://doi.org/10.1176/appi. books.9780890425596.dsm09. See also, above, n. 25 to ch. 3.
7. Cynthia Stonnington et al., 'Conversion and Somatic Symptom Disorders', *BMJ Best Practice*, January 2018, https://bestpractice.bmj.com/topics/en-us/989
8. https://icd.who.int/dev11/f/en#/http%3a%2f%2fid.who.int%2ficd%2fentity%2f1069443471
9. Jon Stone et al., 'Issues for DSM-5: Conversion Disorder', *American Journal of Psychiatry* 167: 6, June 2010, pp. 626–7. See also, American Psychiatric Association Division of Research, 'Highlights of Changes from DSM-IV to DSM-5: Somatic Symptom and Related Disorders', *Focus: Psychosomatic Medicine and Integrated Care*, 11: 4, Fall 2013, pp. 525–7, https://focus.psychiatryonline.org/doi/10.1176/appi. focus.11.4.525
10. The notion of 'flight, fright, freeze' is by now a widespread notion, a popular way of understanding stress, trauma, anxiety and so on. See David S. Goldstein, 'Adrenal Responses to Stress', *Cellular and Molecular Biology*, 30: 8, 2010, pp. 1,433–40. As Goldstein writes, physiologist Walter Cannon, in the 1920s, was the first to describe 'the acute changes in adrenal gland secretion associated with what he called "fight or flight" responses'. These happened in response to threats to what Cannon had termed 'homeostasis', his coinage 'to describe the maintenance within acceptable ranges of physiological variables such as blood glucose and core temperature'. For a study of the neural mechanisms involved in freezing, see Karin Roelofs, 'Freeze For Action: Neurobiological Mechanisms in Animal and Human Freezing', *Philosophical Transactions of the Royal Society B*, 372: 1718, 19 April 2017.
11. Selma Aybek et al., 'Emotion–Motion Interactions in Conversion Disorder: An fMRI Study', *PLoS One*, 10: 4, 10 April 2015: there is 'significantly increased activation . . . in areas involved in the "freeze response" to fear (periaqueductal grey matter), and areas involved in self-awareness and motor

control (cingulate gyrus and supplementary motor area).' This would mean that people such as Claire 'exhibited increased response amplitude to fearful stimuli over time, suggesting abnormal emotional regulation'. Their 'activated midbrain and frontal structures', moreover, 'could reflect an abnormal behavioral-motor response to negative including threatening stimuli. This suggests a mechanism linking emotions to motor dysfunction in conversion disorder.'

12. Michel de Montaigne, *The Complete Essays*, trans. M. A. Screech (London and New York, NY: Penguin, 1991), Book 1: 21, 'Of the Power of the Imagination', p. 109.

13. See Fabrizio Benedetti, 'Placebo Effects: From the Neurobiological Paradigm to Translational Implications', *Neuron*, 84: 3, 5 November 2014, pp. 623–37. See also Steve Silberman, 'Placebos Are Getting More Effective. Drugmakers Are Desperate to Know Why', *Wired*, 24 August 2009, https://www.wired.com/2009/08/ff-placebo-effect/. And see my *Passions and Tempers*, pp. 291–5.

14. See Hans-Peter Kapfhammer, 'Somatic Symptoms in Depression', *Dialogues in Clinical Neuroscience*, 8: 2, June 2006, pp. 227–39.

15. See Damasio, *The Feeling of What Happens*, pp. 56–62.

16. See n. 7 above.

17. See Anna Ciaunica, Jane Charlton, and Harry Farmer, 'When the Window Cracks: Transparency and the Fractured Self in Depersonalisation', *Phenomenology and the Cognitive Sciences*, June 2020.

18. Ed Yong, 'COVID-19 Can Last for Several Months', *The Atlantic*, 4 June 2020: 'Such conditions include ME/CFS, fibromyalgia, and postural orthostatic tachycardia syndrome. They disproportionately affect women; have unclear causes, complex but debilitating symptoms, and no treatments; and are hard to diagnose and easy to dismiss. According to the Institute of Medicine, 836,000 to 2.5 million people in the U.S. alone have ME/CFS. Between 84 and 91 percent are undiagnosed.'

19. Stephan Zipfel et al., 'Psychosomatic Medicine in Germany: More Timely than Ever', *Psychotherapy and Psychosomatics*, 85, 2016, pp. 262–9.

20. Hustvedt, *The Shaking Woman*, p. 73.

21. See Mark Solms and Michael Saling, trans. and eds, *A Moment of Transition: Two Neuroscientific Articles by Sigmund Freud* (London and New York, NY: Karnak Books, 1990). The texts are 'Gehirn' and 'Aphasie'.

22. See Makari, *Revolution in Mind*, pp. 30–4.

23. Freud and Breuer, *Studies in Hysteria*, p. 18.

24. See my *Passions and Tempers*, p. 88.

25. See Sander L. Gilman et al., *Hysteria Beyond Freud*, and, above, n. 14 to ch. 2.

26. See Michel de Certeau, *The Possession at Loudun*, trans. Michael B. Smith (Oxford: Blackwells, 2000), and which includes a physician's testimony asserting devilry was at work, pp. 119–21.

27. Roy Porter, *Flesh in the Age of Reason: How the Enlightenment Transformed the Way We See Our Bodies and Souls* (London and New York: Penguin, 2003): 'By the eighteenth century, hysteria, which had earlier been judged a somatic malady of women – a disease of the womb – was typically deployed to identify the volatile physical symptoms associated with hypersensitivity, a lability thought especially common in "the sex", but – significantly, in a culture in which enlightened politeness was blamed for making men "effeminate" – not exclusively so. The diagnosis signalled superiority in status, while also marking a mysterious *je ne sais quoi*, a malady that was intermittent and unpredictable, lacking tangible physical causes . . . This "coming-out" of the hypochondriac and hysteric constitutes an important symptom, the pathological downside of Enlightenment individualism' (pp. 401–2).

28. Charles Lepois, *Selectiorum observationem et consiliorum de praetervisis hactenus morbis* (Ponte ad Monticulum: Carolum Mercatorum, 1618).

29. Thomas Willis, *Cerebri anatome: cui accessit nervorum descriptio et usus* (London, 1664).

30. J. M. S. Pearce, 'Sydenham on Hysteria', *European Neurology*, 76, 2016, pp. 175–81, and which gives the full text of the letter. And see E. Trillat, 'Conversion Disorder and Hysteria: Clinical Section', in Berrios and Porter, *A History of Clinical Psychiatry*, p. 435.

31. Pierre Hunauld, *Dissertation sur les vapeurs et les pertes de sang* (published posthumously in 1756), in Sabine Arnaud, ed., *La Philosophie des vapeurs* (Paris: Mercure de France, 2009).

32. Trillat, in Berrios and Porter, *A History of Clinical Psychiatry*, p. 435. And see R. K. French, *Robert Whytt, The Soul, and Medicine* (London: Wellcome Institute of the History of Medicine, 1969), passim: pp. 31–45.

33. See n. 3 to ch. 2, above.

34. See my *Passions and Tempers*, pp. 249–53.

35. Mark J. Edwards, Aikaterini Fotopoulou, and Isabel Pareés, 'Neurobiology of Functional (Psychogenic) Movement Disorders', *Current Opinion in Neurology*, 26: 4, August 2013, pp. 442–7. See also n. 19 to ch. 2, above; and Bell et al., 'What is the Functional/Organic Distinction Actually Doing in Psychiatry and Neurology?' (2020).

36. William James, 'What is an Emotion?', *Mind*, 9: 34, April 1884, pp. 188–205.

37. A good account of the stress response is Constantine Tsigos et al., 'Stress, Endocrine Physiology and Pathophysiology', *Endotext*, March 2016. And see Bessel van der Kolk, *The Body Keeps the Score: Mind, Brain and Body in the Transformation of Trauma* (New York, NY and London: Penguin, 2014).

38. See Damasio, *The Strange Order of Things*, pp. 82–116.

39. T. R. Nicholson et al., 'Life Events and Escape in Conversion Disorder', *Psychological Medicine*, 46: 12, September 2016, pp. 2,617–26.

40. On narrative as being central to the dialogical self, originating as sensorimotor, pre-linguistic rhythm even *in utero*, see Siri

Hustvedt, 'Pace, Space and the Other in the Making of Fiction', *Costellazioni*, 2: 5, 2018, pp. 23–50.

41. See Kasia Kozlowska et al., 'Fear and the Defense Cascade: Clinical Implications and Management', *Harvard Review of Psychiatry*, 23 :4, July/August 2015, pp. 263–87: 'In evolutionary terms the responses that make up the defense cascade are primitive emotional states – coordinated patterns of motor-autonomic-sensory response – that are available to be automatically activated in the context of danger. Emotions are played out "in the theatre of the body"' (p. 264). The expression quoted here is Damasio's: 'For humans, the activation of defense responses – the sudden change in motor and physiological state – may be experienced as overwhelming, and beyond conscious control' (*Looking for Spinoza*, p. 28).

42. See Joyce McDougall, *Theaters of the Body: A Psychoanalytic Approach to Psychosomatic Illness* (New York, NY: W. W. Norton, 1989).

43. In my 'The Interoceptive Turn' (2019). See also Martin P. Paulus, Justin S. Feinstein, and Sahib S. Khalsa, 'An Active Inference Approach to Interoceptive Psychopathology', *Annual Review of Clinical Psychology*, 2019, 15, pp. 97–122, for a definition of interoception as 'the process by which the nervous system senses, interprets, and integrates signals originating from within the body, provides organisms with a momentary mapping of the body's internal landscape and its relationship to the outside world,' ensuring the body's homeostatic regulation within a constantly changing environment (pp. 98, 115).

44. See Sarah N. Garfinkel, Jessica A. Eccles, and Hugo D. Critchley, 'The Heart, the Brain, and the Regulation of Emotion', *JAMA Psychiatry*, 72: 11, November 2015; Hugo D. Critchley and Sarah N. Garfinkel, 'Interoception and Emotion', *Current Opinion in Psychology*, 17, 2017, pp. 7–14.

45. Feldman Barrett et al., 'An Active Inference Theory of Allostasis and Interoception in Depression': 'primary interoceptive cortex (in the dorsal mid to posterior insula) is a

component of the salience network, ensuring that every mental event (not just emotions) is infused with interoception, which is made available to consciousness as affect' (p. 7).

46. Ana Tajadura-Jiménez, Helen Cohen, and Nadia Bianchi-Berthouze, 'Bodily Sensory Inputs and Anomalous Bodily Experiences in Complex Regional Pain Syndrome: Evaluation of the Potential Effects of Sound Feedback', *Frontiers in Human Neuroscience*, 11: 379, 27 July 2017.

47. Matthew Botvinick and Jonathan Cohen, 'Rubber Hands "Feel" Touch that Eyes See', *Nature*, 391, 19 February 1998, p. 756.

48. Tsakiris, 'The Multisensory Basis of the Self', (2017), pp. 597–609: p. 599. See also my 'The Interoceptive Turn' (2019).

49. Tajadura-Jiménez, Cohen, and Bianchi-Berthouze, 'Bodily Sensory Inputs and Anomalous Bodily Experiences' (2017): 'Previous works have described that some people with CRPS have referred sensations (i.e., the perception of a stimulus at a location distant from the stimulated body site). These sensations are thought to be a clinical correlate of the cortical reorganization found in neuroimaging, psychophysical and transcranial magnetic stimulation studies in areas of the primary and secondary somatosensory cortex responsible for the representation of the affected limb. There is also clinical evidence that in people with CRPS there can be dysfunction of parietal regions. These regions overlap with multisensory parietal areas integrating somatosensory, visual and auditory signals to form mental body representations.'

50. Tsakiris, 'The Multisensory Basis of the Self' (2017).

51. David L. Perez et al., 'A Neural Circuit Framework for Somatosensory Amplification in Somatoform Disorders', *Journal of Neuropsychiatry and Clinical Neurosciences*, 27, Winter 2015, pp. e40–50: p. e40. They write: 'Somatosensory amplification may involve a bidirectional pattern of insula and amygdala activity. Patients with somatization disorder, undifferentiated somatoform disorder, and somatoform pain disorder exhibit insula and amygdala hypoactivity to external (environmental) emotionally valenced stimuli. Amygdalar and

insular hypoactivity was also observed in subjects with alexithymia exposed to extrinsic emotionally valenced stimuli. Conversely, delivery of self-oriented, bodily-related stimuli (i.e., tactile) increased amygdala and insula activity in patients with somatoform pain disorder, and these regions also showed hyperactivity in studies of negative attentional bias. These findings suggest that somatosensory amplification may be partially the result of selective heightened attention and salience for bodily sensations (internal states) and parallel under-processing of external emotionally valenced information' (p. e45).

52. See Georg Northoff, *Neuro-Philosophy and the Healthy Mind: Learning from the Unwell Brain* (New York, NY and London: W. W. Norton, 2016), pp. 86–114.

53. See Valerie Voon et al., 'Aberrant Supplementary Motor Complex and Limbic Activity During Motor Preparation in Motor Conversion Disorder', *Movement Disorders*, 26: 13, November 2011, pp. 2,396–403: 'Conversion disorder (CD) is characterized by unexplained neurological symptoms presumed related to psychological issues. The main hypotheses to explain conversion paralysis, characterized by a lack of movement, include impairments in either motor intention or disruption of motor execution, and further, that hyperactive self-monitoring, limbic processing or top-down regulation from higher order frontal regions may interfere with motor execution . . . We propose a theory in which previously mapped conversion motor representations may in an arousing context hijack the voluntary action selection system, which is both hypoactive and functionally disconnected from prefrontal top-down regulation' (abstract). See also Yann Cojanet et al., 'Motor Inhibition in Hysterical Conversion Paralysis', *Neuroimage*, 47: 3, September 2009, for a study of motor and inhibitory brain circuits which suggests 'that conversion symptoms do not act through cognitive inhibitory circuits, but involve selective activations in midline brain regions associated with self-related representations and emotion regulation' (abstract).

54. Carlo Cavaliere et al., 'Microstructural Changes in Motor Functional Conversion Disorder: Multimodal Imaging Approach on a Case', *Brain Sciences*, 10: 385, June 2020: 'To ascertain the absence of organic lesions, neuroimaging techniques are largely used. In a study by Voon et al., patients with motor conversion tremor exhibited a reduced functional connectivity between the temporo-parietal junction and the sensorimotor and limbic regions during the involuntary tremor but not during the voluntary reproduction of their conversion tremor, suggesting a lack of self-agency as a core feature in conversion disorder. Conversely, Aybek et al., "Emotion–Motion Interactions" (2015), found in patients with motor conversion disorder increased activity in the supplementary motor area (SMA) and in limbic areas associated with emotional processing during motor preparation and inhibition, self-initiated action and sense of agency. Moreover, the authors examining patients with motor conversion disorder observed a greater amygdala and frontal network activity in response to negative emotional stimuli, suggesting an abnormal crosstalk between emotion and motion areas. Several examinations using positron emission tomography (PET) have showed hypermetabolism in the frontal areas, explained as the result of active inhibition of the sensorimotor area that translates into limb paralysis; hypermetabolism in the cerebellum and basal ganglia; and an opposite pattern of reduced blood flow in the primary motorcortex.'

55. Paulus et al., 'An Active Inference Approach to Interoceptive Psychopathology', pp. 103–4, p. 110: 'these dysfunctions [of somatic symptoms] are best understood as the result of a persistent discrepancy between a model that generates strong expectations of an aversive interoceptive percept and evidence that is at odds with this expectation, together with an inability of the prediction error to adjust the model' (p. 110).

56. See Pitron et al., 'Troubles somatiques fonctionnels': 'La pérennisation de symptomes physiques dans les troubles

somatiques fonctionnels semble procéder d'une prophétie auto-réalisatrice: ils surviennent justement parce qu'ils sont anticipés par le cerveau. La prédiction cognitive que le symptôme va resurgir n'est pas en elle-même un processus dont le patient peut prendre conscience et qu'il peut contrôler. Elle est favorisée par une réaction émotionnelle particulièrement intense lors d'un épisode inaugural intercurrent' (p. 468).

57. The idea has been developed notably in Mark J. Edwards et al., 'A Bayesian Account of 'Hysteria', *Brain*, 135: 11, November 2012, pp. 3,495–512.

58. Seth and Tsakiris, 'Being a Beast Machine' (2018), pp. 969–81: p. 974.

59. See Fabienne Picard and Karl Friston, 'Predictions, Perception, and a Sense of Self', *Neurology*, 83, 16 September 2014, pp. 1,112–18.

60. See Valerie Voon et al., 'The Involuntary Nature of Conversion Disorder', *Neurology*, 74: 3, 19 January 2010, pp. 223–8. In conversion patients, 'the perception that the conversion movement is not self-generated' is associated with lower activity in the right temporoparietal junction, an area of the brain that 'has been implicated as a general comparator of internal predictions with actual events', and with fewer interactions of that area with the sensorimotor cortex.

61. See Daniel M. Wolpert and J. Randall Flanagan, 'Motor Prediction', *Current Biology*, 11: 18. The notion of efference copy was developed over the 1950s within work on visual perception notably by Erich von Holst and Roger Sperry, on the basis of an idea first mooted by German physicist Hermann von Helmholtz in the mid-nineteenth century. See Bruce Bridgeman, 'How the Brain Makes the World Appear Stable', *Iperception*, 1: 2, November 2010, pp. 69–72.

62. Edwards, Fotopolou, and Pareés, 'Neurobiology of Functional (Psychogenic) Movement Disorders' (2013): 'The key concept here is of a "previously mapped conversion motor representation", that is, a (conditioned) pattern of movement

established perhaps by a previous triggering event. The commonly reported presence of physical precipitating factors at onset such as injury could provide a relevant trigger for development of a "conversion motor representation". The additional emotional arousal that is often reported in the background and/or at the time of onset could certainly increase the salience of sensory information arising during a physical trigger and facilitate this process. Functional imaging studies from this group have provided evidence for hypoactivity in areas usually associated with action selection (e.g., supplementary motor area (SMA)), as well as abnormally strong connectivity between limbic structures (e.g., amygdala) and SMA (26,28). The proposal is that in an arousing context, the previously mapped conversion motor representation is activated in part because of the abnormal functional connectivity between limbic structures and SMA, and cannot be inhibited because there is a disconnection between SMA and areas (prefrontal cortex for example) that could usually inhibit unwanted action. The result is a movement that arises without a normal prediction of its sensory consequences (efference copy) and is therefore (mis)interpreted by patients as without agency and therefore not self-generated.'

63. See Sarah-Jayne Blakemore, Daniel Wolpert, and Chris Frith, 'Why Can't You Tickle Yourself?', *NeuroReport*, 11: 11, 3 August 2000. See also Anouk van der Weiden, Merel Prikken, and Neeltje E. M. van Haren, 'Self–Other Integration and Distinction in Schizophrenia: A Theoretical Analysis and a Review of the Evidence', *Neuroscience & Biobehavioral Reviews*, 57, October 2015, pp. 220–37: 'Compared with healthy controls, schizophrenia patients report stronger rubber hand illusions. This supports the notion that patients have a more flexible representation of their "self", resulting in a reduced ability to distinguish self and other and a tendency to over-attribute external events or objects (such as a rubber hand) to themselves' (p. 223).

64. See Selma Aybek et al., 'Neural Correlates of Recall of Life

Events in Conversion Disorder', *JAMA Psychiatry*, 71: 1, January 2014. The way in which 'adverse events are processed cognitively can be associated with physical symptoms': 'Abnormal emotion (dorsolateral prefrontal cortex and right inferior frontal cortex) and memory control (hippocampus) are associated with alterations in symptom-related motor planning and body schema (supplementary motor area and temporoparietal junction) (p. 52).' And see Patrick Haggard and Manos Tsakiris, 'The Experience of Agency: Feelings, Judgments, and Responsibility', *Current Directions in Psychological Science*, 18: 4, 2009, pp. 242–6.

65. Antonio Damasio, 'The Somatic Marker Hypothesis and the Possible Functions of the Prefrontal Cortex', *Philosophical Transactions of the Royal Society B*, 351: 1346, 29 October 1996, pp. 1,413–20. Damasio explains his 'somatic marker hypothesis' as the process of feeling our emotions, that recruits brain regions involved in homeostasis. Without these feelings, we cannot make decisions: 'marker' signals influence the processes of response to stimuli, at multiple levels of operation, some of which occur overtly (consciously, "in mind") and some of which occur covertly (non-consciously, in a non-minded manner). The marker signals arise in bioregulatory processes, including those which express themselves in emotions and feelings, but are not necessarily confined to those alone. This is the reason why the markers are termed somatic: they relate to body-state structure and regulation even when they do not arise in the body proper but rather in the brain's representation of the body' (abstract). As I wrote in 'The Interoceptive Turn' (2019): 'We don't merely think through our decisions, including those that seem most rational, such as those concerning finances: we experience feelings about their possible outcomes that determine how we act – and if the brain areas involved in the processing of emotional feelings are damaged, our ability to make decisions is impaired.'

66. Kozlowska et al., 'Fear and the Defense Cascade', p. 279. And see Lisa Quadt, Hugo D. Critchley, and Sarah N. Garfinkel,

'The Neurobiology of Interoception in Health and Disease', *Annals of the New York Academy of Sciences*, 1428: 1, September 2018, pp. 112–28.

67. Tajadura-Jiménez, Cohen, and Bianchi-Berthouze, 'Bodily Sensory Inputs and Anomalous Bodily Experiences' (2017).

68. Daniele di Lernia et al., 'Altered Interoceptive Perception and the Effects of Interoceptive Analgesia in Musculoskeletal, Primary, and Neuropathic Chronic Pain Conditions', *Journal of Personalized Medicine*, 10: 4, 2020. Acknowledging that 'pain is a complex pathological condition that poorly responds to pain management treatments and therapies', the authors devised 'a novel potential interoceptive treatment for CP [Chronic Pain], using a non-invasive method to induce analgesia through interoceptive stimulation of the C-Tactile afferents in the skin' (p. 12). They write in the abstract: 'As pain is inherently an interoceptive signal, interoceptive frameworks provide important, but underutilized, approaches to this condition', hence their treatment, using affective touch, to activate 'the C-Tactile system, by means of controlled stimulation of interoceptive unmyelinated afferents'. This 'led to significant pain reduction (mean 23%) in the CP treatment group after only 11 min.' See also Bruno Muller-Oerlinghausen and Michael Eggart, eds., *The Significance of Touch in Psychiatry: Clinical and Neuroscientific Approaches* (Basel: MDPI, 2021).

69. Mark Solms, 'The Neurobiological Underpinnings of Psychoanalytic Theory and Therapy', *Frontiers in Behavioral Neuroscience*, 4 December 2018.

70. See David Sumasy, 'Diseases and Natural Kinds', *Theoretical Medicine and Bioethics*, 26: 6, December 2005, pp. 487–513.

Chapter 8: Impostors

1. See Andrea Scalabrini et al., 'Dissociation as a Disorder of Integration – On the Footsteps of Pierre Janet', *Progress in Neuropsychopharmacology and Biological Psychiatry*, 101, 2020.

2. See Ciaunica, Charlton, and Farmer, 'When the Window Cracks' (2020), https://aeon.co/essays/what-can-depersonalisation-disorder-say-about-the-self.

3. Canguilhem, *Le Normal et le pathologique*, p. 155. See also, above, n. 24 to ch. 1.

4. See Daniel B. Auerbach, 'The Ganser Syndrome', in Claude T. H. Friedmann and Robert A. Faguet, eds, *Extraordinary Disorders of Human Behavior* (Springer, 2012).

5. Walther Riese and A. Requet, 'L'Etat crépusculaire hystérique (Ganser)', *L'Encéphale*, 32, 1937, pp. 209–26.

6. The term pseudo-dementia was first coined some sixty years ago by Leslie Kiloh, in relation to Ganser Syndrome: 'Pseudo-Dementia', *Acta Psychiatrica Scandinavica*, December 1961. See also John Snowdon, 'Pseudodementia, a Term for Its Time: The Impact of Leslie Kiloh's 1961 Paper', *Australasian Psychiatry*, 19: 5, October 2011, pp. 391–7.

7. Paolo Scopelliti and Roger Dadoun, *L'Influence du surréalisme sur la psychanalyse* (Paris: L'Age d'Homme, 2002), p. 28.

8. Sebastian Dieguez, 'Ganser Syndrome', in Julien Bogousslavsky, ed., *Neurologic-Psychiatric Syndromes in Focus – Part II: From Psychiatry to Neurology* (Basel: Karger, 2018), Frontiers of Neurology and Neuroscience, 42, pp. 1–22.

9. Munchausen Syndrome is also known as 'factitious disorder imposed on self' (it can also be 'imposed on another'), and features in the *DSM 5* under 'somatic disorders'. See Muhammad Zeshan, Raminder Cheema, and Pankaj Manocha, 'Challenges in Diagnosing Factitious Disorder', *American Journal of Psychiatry*, 13: 9, 1 September 2018, pp. 6–8.

10. H. W. Lebourgeois, 'Malingering: Key Points in Assessment', *Psychiatric Times*, 15 April 2007. See also Riese and Requet, 'L'Etat crépusculaire hystérique (Ganser), (1937), p. 225.

11. Auerbach, 'The Ganser Syndrome', in Friedmann and Faguet, eds, *Extraordinary Disorders of Human Behavior*, p. 44. The psychiatrist and philosopher Karl Jaspers discussed this phenomenon at length in his *Allgemeine Psychopathologie*, first

published in 1913: see *General Psychopathology*, vol. 2 (Baltimore, MD: Johns Hopkins University Press, 1997), p. 593.

12. Daniel Ouyang, Harpreet S. Duggal, and N. J. Jacob, 'Neurological Basis of Ganser Syndrome', *Indian Journal of Psychiatry*, 45: 4, 2003, pp. 255–6.

13. Eloi Magnin et al., 'Conversion, Dissociative Amnesia, and Ganser Syndrome in a Case of '"Chameleon" Syndrome: Anatomo-Functional Findings', *Neurocase: The Neural Basis of Cognition*, 20: 1, 2014; also Elsa Kaphan et al., 'Ganser-like Syndrome After Loss of Psychic Self-activation Syndrome: Psychogenic or Organic?' *Archives of Clinical Neuropsychology*, 29: 7, November 2014, pp. 715–23.

14. Riese and Requet, 'L'Etat crépusculaire' (1937), p. 220.

15. See under 'Dissociative Disorders', in the *Diagnostic and Statistical Manual of Mental Disorders*, 5th edition (American Psychiatric Association, 2013), https://dsm.psychiatryonline. org/doi/10.1176/appi.books.9780890425596.dsm08, and for the *ICD* entry, see https://icd.codes/icd10cm/F4481

16. Ian Hacking's *Rewriting the Soul: Multiple Personality and the Science of Memory* (Princeton, NJ: Princeton University Press, 1995) is an exploration of the epistemology and metaphysics inherent in 'attempts to scientize the soul through the study of memory' (p. 6). See also Numan Gharaibeh, 'Dissociative Identity Disorder: Time to Remove It From DSM-V?', *Current Psychiatry*, 8: 9, September 2009, pp. 30–6.

17. Scalabrini et al., 'Dissociation as a Disorder of Integration' (2020), p. 2, and the quotation is from Pierre Janet, *The Major Symptoms of Hysteria: Fifteen Lectures Given in the Medical School of Harvard University* (London and New York, NY: Macmillan, 1907).

18. For a view that the syndrome is less rare than is usually deemed, see Bethany L. Brand et al., 'Separating Fact from Fiction: An Empirical Examination of Six Myths About Dissociative Identity Disorder', *Harvard Review of Psychiatry*, 24: 4, July 2016, pp. 257–70.

19. Yasufumi Tanaka et al., 'Diagonistic Dyspraxia: Clinical Characteristics, Responsible Lesion and Possible Underlying Mechanism', *Brain*, 119: 3, 1996, pp. 859–74.
20. See Hacking, *Rewriting the Soul*: 'One person, one soul, may have many facets and speak with many souls' (p. 6).
21. See Aybek et al., 'Emotion–Motion Interactions in Conversion Disorder' (2015), and n. 9 to ch. 7 above. The authors report: 'We found increased amygdala activation to negative emotions in CD compared to healthy controls in region of interest analyses, which persisted over time consistent with previous findings using emotional paradigms. Furthermore during whole brain analyses we found significantly increased activation in CD patients in areas involved in the "freeze response" to fear (periaqueductal grey matter), and areas involved in self-awareness and motor control (cingulate gyrus and supplementary motor area).'
22. John Bowlby, *Attachment* (London: Tavistock Institute of Human Relations, 1969/New York, NY: Basic Books, 1982).
23. See Samantha Reisz, Robbie Duschinsky, and Daniel J. Siegel, 'Disorganized Attachment and Defense: Exploring John Bowlby's Unpublished Reflections', *Attachment and Human Development*, 20: 2, 2018, pp. 107–34. And see Daniel J. Siegel, *The Developing Mind: How Relationships and the Brain Interact to Shape Who We Are*, 3rd edition (New York, NY: Guilford Press, 2020).
24. See van der Kolk, *The Body Keeps the Score*, pp. 184–99.
25. On the stress response, see, above, n. 35 to ch. 7.
26. Anna Ciaunica has been conducting research on the phenomenon: see n. 2 above. And see Alexandre Billon, 'Mineness First: Three Challenges to the Recent Theories of the Sense of Bodily Ownership', in de Vignemont and Alsmith, eds, *The Subject's Matter*, pp. 189–216, and his argument that 'mineness' is a 'primitive' phenomenon that 'cannot be accounted for in psychological terms', whether these appeal to 'sensory, interoceptive, sensorimotor, or affective dispositions' (p. 210).

27. Hacking, *Rewriting the Soul*. What was important about Ribot and scientists like him, writes Hacking, 'was not that they had a program but that they offered knowledge' precisely about a hard-to-grasp entity that, at the time at least, escaped a neurological account of the mind. Hacking contrasts this stance with our modern belief that the truth of ourself lies somewhere precise, indeed that there is such a thing as a true self at all (p. 208).

28. Ibid.

29. James, *The Principles of Psychology*, vol. 1, ch. 10, 'The Consciousness of Self', pp. 279–313.

30. See, above, n. 3 to ch. 3.

31. See Giuseppe Riva, 'The Neuroscience of Body Memory: From the Self Through the Space to the Others', *Cortex*, 104, 2018, pp. 241–60: 'the contents of the body matrix are modified by bottom-up prediction errors that signal mismatches between predicted and actual content of the different body representations. An important effect of this process is the top-down modulation induced by multisensory conflicts over the contents of the different body representations, starting from the first one, i.e., The Sentient Body, which has direct access to the interoceptive homeostatic systems' (p. 500). See also Tsakiris, 'The Multisensory Basis of the Self' (2017).

32. Edmund Husserl, the founder of phenomenology, distinguished the physical *Körper* from the experiencing *Leib*. See Maren Wehrle, 'Being a Body and Having a Body: The Twofold Temporality of Embodied Intentionality', *Phenomenology and the Cognitive Sciences*, 2019.

Chapter 9: The Affront

1. See Cory Toth, 'Hemisensory Syndrome is Associated with a Low Diagnostic Yield and a Nearly Uniform Benign Prognosis', *Journal of Neurology, Neurosurgery & Psychiatry*, 74: 8, 2003, pp. 1,113–16.

2. See Paul Guyer and Allen Wood, Introduction to their translation and edition of Immanuel Kant, *Critique of Pure Reason* (1781) (Cambridge and New York, NY: Cambridge University Press, 1998),: 'space and time are neither subsistent beings nor inherent in things as they are in themselves, but are rather only forms of our sensibility, hence conditions under which objects of experience can be given at all and the fundamental principle of their representation and individuation' (p. 7).

3. John Locke, *An Essay Concerning Human Understanding* (1690) (Oxford: Clarendon Press, 1979), ed. Peter H. Nidditch, Book 2, ch. 27, 'Of Identity and Diversity'.

4. David Hume, *A Treatise of Human Nature: Being an Attempt to introduce the experimental Method of Reasoning into Moral Subjects* (London, 1739), Book 1, Part 4.

5. Northoff, *Neuro-Philosophy and the Healthy Mind*, p. 183.

6. James, *The Principles of Psychology*, vol. 1, p. 574.

7. Ibid., p. 603.

8. Ibid., p. 593.

9. See above, n. 28 and n. 29 to ch. 3.

10. Wittmann and Meissner, 'The Embodiment of Time' in Tsakiris and de Preester, eds, *The Interoceptive Mind*, pp. 63–79: 'subjective time emerges only through the existence of the self across time as an enduring and embodied entity' (p. 64).

11. Ibid.: such patients, write Wittmann and Meissner, feel 'a detachment from their own bodies', along with 'disturbances in the subjective sense of time that are complemented by impairments in objective timing tasks' (p. 75). See also Ciaunica, Charlton, and Farmer, 'When the Window Cracks' (2020), and Harry Farmer et al, 'The Detached Self: Investigating the Effect of Depersonalisation on Self-bias in the Visual Remapping of Touch', *Multisensory Research*, October 2020. See also Alexandre Billon, 'Making Sense of the Cotard Syndrome: Insights from the Study of Depersonalisation', *Mind & Language*, 31: 3, June 2016, pp. 356–91.

12. Wittmann and Meissner, 'The Embodiment of Time' in Tsakiris and de Preester, eds, *The Interoceptive Mind*, p. 66.

13. A. D. (Bud) Craig, 'How Do You Feel? Interoception: The Sense of the Physiological Condition of the Body', *Nature Reviews Neuroscience*, 3, 2002, pp. 655–66. Craig detailed 'an afferent neural system in primates and in humans that represents all aspects of the physiological condition of the physical body. This system constitutes a representation of "'the material me", and might provide a foundation for subjective feelings, emotion and self-awareness' (abstract). Craig identified the interoceptive pathways that provide a cortical image of homeostatic processes from all the organs, and which translate as feelings when brought to consciousness. See A. D. (Bud) Craig, *How Do You Feel? An Interoceptive Moment with Your Neurobiological Self* (Princeton, NJ: Princeton University Press, 2014): Craig and his team individuated projections to the brainstem of neurons in the spinal cord called lamina I. These provide to the autonomic nervous system input about the 'mechanical, thermal, chemical, metabolic and hormonal status of skin, muscle, joints, teeth and viscera' from small-diameter nerves throughout the organism's tissues. It is from these lamina I projections to brainstem that 'sensory channels' ascend to areas of the thalamus, and from there to the insula, often nicknamed the 'interoceptive cortex' (p. 500).

14. A. D. (Bud) Craig, 'Emotional Moments Across Time: A Possible Neural Basis for Time Perception in the Anterior Insula', *Philosophical Transactions of The Royal Society B*, 364: 1525, 2009, pp. 1,933–42: p. 1,932.

15. For an analysis of this 'material me' and of how 'interoception serves the unity and stability of the self', see Manos Tsakiris, 'The Material Me: Unifying the Exteroceptive and Interoceptive Sides of the Bodily Self', in de Vignemont and Alsmith, eds, *The Subject's Matter*, pp. 335–61.

16. See above, n. 42 to ch. 7. And see Sarah G. Garfinkel et al., 'Interoceptive Dimensions Across Cardiac and Respiratory

Axes', *Philosophical Transactions of the Royal Society B*, 371: 1708, November 2016. The value of heartbeat detection tasks has been critiqued recently: see in particular Giorgia Zamariola et al., 'Interoceptive Accuracy Scores from the Heartbeat Counting Task are Problematic: Evidence from Simple Bivariate Correlations', *Biological Psychology*, 137, September 2018, pp. 12–17. Discussions are ongoing regarding the possible methodologies for gauging accurately levels of interoceptive accuracy, sensibility, and awareness. On these latter distinctions, see Sarah N. Garfinkel et al., 'Knowing Your Own Heart: Distinguishing Interoceptive Accuracy from Interoceptive Awareness', *Biological Psychology*, 104, January 2015, pp. 65–74.

17. See an analysis of such studies by Karin Meissner and Marc Wittmann, 'Body Signals, Cardiac Awareness, and the Perception of Time', *Biological Psychology*, 86: 3, March 2011, pp. 289–97.

18. See Olga Pollatos et al., 'How Much Time Has Passed? Ask Your Heart', *Frontiers in Neurorobotics*, 9 April 2014. The authors cite in their introduction Craig's contention in his 2009 paper (see n. 14 above) that 'the neural substrates responsible for sentience across time are based on the neural representation of the physiological condition of the body, and that the main homeostatic (autonomic) control function for the maintenance of the physiological condition of the body is cardiorespiratory activity,' and in effect show this is the case.

19. See Sarah N. Garfinkel et al., 'Fear from the Heart: Sensitivity to Fear Stimuli Depends on Individual Heartbeats', *Journal of Neuroscience*, 34: 19, May 2014, pp. 6,573–82. See also Richard D. Lane et al., 'Neural Correlates of Heart Rate Variability During Emotion', *Neuroimage*, 44: 1, January 2009, pp. 213–22.

20. See Wittmann and Meissner, 'The Embodiment of Time' in Tsakiris and de Preester, eds, *The Interoceptive Mind*: for instance, 'impulsivity can be understood as a strongly felt urge for immediate gratification, which is generated through the interoceptive system' (p. 69).

21. Karl Friston and Gyorgy Buzsáki, 'The Functional Anatomy of Time: What and When in the Brain', *Trends in Cognitive Sciences*, 20: 7, July 2016, pp. 500–11. The authors apply Friston's notion of how, when one considers the brain in Bayesian terms, 'the structure of a good brain will recapitulate the (statistical) structure of how sensations are caused' (p. 501).

22. György Buzsáki and Rodolfo Llinás, 'Space and Time in the Brain', *Science*, 358, October 2017, pp. 482–5 and Rodolfo Llinás, in his *I of the Vortex: From Neurons to Self* (Cambridge, MA and London: MIT Press, 2001) defines the self as 'the centralization of prediction'.

23. Buszáki and Llinás, 'Space and Time in the Brain' (2017). The authors write of 'a brain that constructs structured sequences of neuronal cell assemblies whose function is to infer trajectories through the lived or explored world' (p. 1).

24. See Agustín Ibáñez et al., 'Cardiac Interoception in Neurological Conditions and its Relevance for Dimensional Approaches', in Tsakiris and de Preester, eds, *The Interoceptive Mind*, pp. 187–213: p. 196, and Richard J. Stevenson et al., 'Hippocampal Dependent Neuropsychological Tests and their Relationship to Measures of Cardiac and Self-report Interoception', *Brain and Cognition*, 123, June 2018, pp. 23–9.

25. Buszáki and Llinás (2017): 'neural algorithms that support map-based navigation are consonant with those needed to create and remember semantic knowledge' (p. 2).

26. Ibid.: connections between events occur by our 'referencing to and linking cortical areas where semantic details of the events are processed' (p. 3).

Chapter 10: Coda

1. See Edmund T. Rolls, 'The Orbitofrontal Cortex and Emotion in Health and Disease, Including Depression', *Neuropsychologia*, 128, May 2019, pp. 14–43.

2. See Lorenzo Pelizza and Federica Bonazzi, 'What's Happened

to Paraphrenia? A Case-report and Review of the Literature', *Acta bio-medica: Atenei Parmensis*, 81: 2, September 2010, pp. 130–40.

3. Advanced, but maybe not as exceptional as we think: the human brain is just one among many others in the animal world, and part of a continuum of consciousness. We don't know what rabbit or dolphin or crow subjectivity is like, and I know of no animal neuropsychiatry clinic, but we may understand ourselves better in the context of other animals, and live better if we relativize our importance. Thanks to philosopher Emanuele Coccia for a conversation that pierced through the speciesism I thought I had conquered – but hadn't.

4. Hustvedt, 'The Delusions of Certainty', in Hustvedt, *A Woman Looking at Men*, pp. 281–294. See also, above, n. 13 to ch. 1.

5. Thanks to biophysicist Mathieu Coppey for a conversation on this topic.

6. See for instance Luca Passamonti, Claire J. Lansdall, and James B. Rowe, 'The Neuroanatomical and Neurochemical basis of Apathy and Impulsivity in Frontotemporal Lobar Degeneration', *Current Opinion in Behavioral Sciences*, 22, 2018, pp. 14–20.

7. See above, n. 13 and n. 14 to ch. 9.

8. See Antonio Damasio, Hanna Damasio, and Daniel Tranel, 'Persistence of Feelings and Sentience after Bilateral Damage of the Insula', *Cerebral Cortex*, 23, April 2013, pp. 833–46.

9. Galen Strawson, 'Against Narrativity', *Ratio*, 17, 2004, pp. 428–52.

10. Ibid.: 'it seems clear to me, when I am experiencing or apprehending myself as a self, that the remoter past or future in question is not my past or future, although it is certainly the past or future of GS the human being' (p. 433). In Strawson's view, one may have 'autobiographical memories' that have 'a "from-the-inside" character' without it necessarily following that 'I experience them as having happened to me*' – where this me*, or I* is 'that which I now experience myself to be when I'm apprehending myself specifically as an inner mental presence or self.'

11. See above, n. 4 to ch. 9.

12. John Dupré, *Processes of Life: Essays in the Philosophy of Biology* (Oxford and New York, NY: Oxford University Press, 2012).

13. Besides the proteinopathies, vascular dementia is very common, and consists in the accruing of microbleeds that end up affecting cognitive and executive functions, and usually memory processes foremost.

14. See Manos Tsakiris and Hugo Critchley, 'Interoception Beyond Homeostasis: Affect, Cognition and Mental Health', and Indira García-Cordero et al., 'Feeling, Learning From and Being Aware of Inner States: Interoceptive Dimensions in Neurodegeneration and Stroke', both in *Philosophical Transactions of the Royal Society B*, 371: 1708, November 2016. See also James M. Kilner et al., 'Impaired Interoceptive Accuracy in Semantic Variant Primary Progressive Aphasia', *Frontiers in Neurology*, November 2017.

15. See Tsakiris and Critchley, 'Interoception Beyond Homeostasis' (2016).

16. See for instance Damiano Azzalini, Ignacio Rebollo, and Catherine Tallon-Baudry, 'Visceral Signals Shape Brain Dynamics and Cognition', *Trends in Cognitive Sciences*, 23: 6, June 2019, pp. 488–509 and Marilia Carabotti et al., 'The Gut–brain Axis: Interactions Between Enteric Microbiota, Central and Enteric Nervous Systems', *Annals of Gastroenterology*, 28: 2, April–June 2015, pp. 203–9.

Index

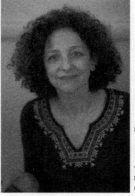

© *Joshua van Praag*

Noga Arikha is a philosopher and historian of ideas. The author of *Passions and Tempers*, she is associate fellow of the Warburg Institute, honorary fellow of the Center for the Politics of Feelings, London, and research associate at the Institut Jean Nicod, Paris. She lives in Florence, Italy.